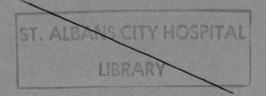

Gastroenterology

IN

PRACTICE

Ian G. Barrison BSc, MB, MRCP

Consultant Physician and Gastroenterologist,
St Albans City and Hemel Hempstead General Hospitals,
Hertfordshire, UK

Michael G. Anderson MD, MRCP

Consultant Physician and Gastroenterologist,
West Middlesex University Hospital,
Isleworth, UK

Peter B. McIntyre MD, MRCP

Consultant Physician and Gastroenterologist,
Queen Elizabeth II Hospital,
Welwyn Garden City,
and Hertford County Hospital, Hertford,
Hertfordshire, UK

Gower Medical Publishing • LONDON • NEW YORK

Distributed in USA and Canada by:
J.B. Lippincott Company
East Washington Square
Philadelphia
PA 19105
USA

Distributed in the UK and Continental Europe by:
Gower Medical Publishing
Middlesex House
34–42 Cleveland Street
London W1P 5FB

Distributed in Australia and New Zealand by:
Harper Educational (Australia) Pty Ltd
PO Box 226
Artarmon
NSW 2064
AUSTRALIA

Distributed in Southeast Asia, Hong Kong and Taiwan by:
APAC Publishers Services
30 Jalan Bahasa
SINGAPORE 1129

Distributed in Japan by:
Nankodo Co Ltd
42-6 Hongo 3-Chome
Bunkyo-ku
Tokyo 113
JAPAN

Distributed in South America by:
HarperCollins Publishers Latin America
701 Bricknell Avenue
Suite 1750
Miami
Florida 33131
USA

Publisher:	Fiona Foley
Project Managers:	Louise Clairmonte Alison Whitehouse
Design and Illustrations:	Anne-Marie Woodruff
Line artist:	Lee Smith
Index:	Nina Boyd
Production:	Susan Bishop

British Library Cataloguing in Publication Data:
Barrison, I.G.
Gastroenterology in practice.
I. Title   II. Anderson, M.G.   III. McIntyre, P.B.
616.30028

Library of Congress Cataloging in Publication Data:
available on request

ISBN 0-379-44788-4

Typeset on Apple Macintosh®
CRC output by the Text Unit
Text set in Garamond; legends set in Futura

Orignated by Chroma Graphics, Singapore

Produced by Mandarin Offset (HK) Ltd, Hong Kong
Printed and bound in Hong Kong

Cover endoscopy: Duodenal ulcer of the
posterior wall, reproduced with kind permission of
Professor Doctor G. N. J. Tytgat, from F. E. Silverstein &
G. N. J. Tytgat, *Atlas of Gastrointestinal Endoscopy*,
2nd edition, Gower Medical Publishing 1991.

Preface

The dramatic advances of the past decade in diagnostic and therapeutic services for gastroenterology justify reappraisal of the family practioner's clinical approach to patients with gastrointestinal problems. This book does not aim to be a comprehensive guide to all aspects of gastroenterology, but instead has focused down on the most common problems presenting in family practice.

Chapters take a common-sense approach to the clinical history, diagnostic techniques and the most appropriate forms of treatment. Recent advances, particularly in the areas of therapeutic endoscopy and in investigation of liver disease, are highlighted, and each chapter contains 'points to remember' which should allow the most appropriate forms of management to be considered.

We do not apologise for including chapters on functional bowel disease or for the apparent emphasis on peptic ulceration and reflux oesophagitis as, in general practice, these problems account for up to two-thirds of consultations for gastroenterological disease.

Whilst not attempting to be didactic, the advice we hope is typical of that offered by practising gastroenterologists working in busy general hospitals. We hope that you find this a useful reference, and also that the illustrations and format of the book allow an enjoyable read.

IAN G. BARRISON
MICHAEL G. ANDERSON
PETER B. McINTYRE

Dedication and Acknowledgements

We dedicate this book to our colleagues at the West Middlesex and Charing Cross Hospitals and in particular to Doctors Jimmy Stewart and Tony Parkins. We are also grateful to our long-suffering families and secretaries for their forbearance and support in the preparation of the text.

We would like to thank the following for providing illustrative material:
The Celiac Society (Fig. 4.14), Dr R. Dick (Fig. 4.15), Dr E. Harder (Figs 1.20, 3.5a); Dr I. N. McNeil, Ealing Hospital, Uxbridge (Figs 4.6, 4.20, 5.6, 6.10, 8.6b, 9.8–9.15, 9.21–9.24, 9.26–9.30, 10.6–10.9); Dr J. J. Misiewicz, Central Middlesex Hospital, London, Dr C. I. Bartram, St Mark's and St Bartholemew's Hospitals, London, Professor P. B. Cotton, Duke University Medical Center, North Carolina, Dr A. S. Mee, The Battle Hospital, Reading, Dr A. B. Price, Northwick Park Hospital, Harrow, and Dr R. P. H. Thompson, St Thomas' Hospital, London (Figs 2.6, 2.7, 2.10, 2.11, 2.19–2.21, 4.2, 4.3, 4.7, 4.10–4.13, 4.18, 4.21, 5.7, 5.8, 5.16–5.18, 6.15, 6.17, 6.19, 6.20, 8.3, 8.7b, 8.9b, 8.12, 8.13, 8.16, 9.35); Professor F. A. Mitros, University of Iowa Hospital, Iowa City (Fig. 5.5); Dr J. Newman (Fig. 5.13); Dr D. Nolan (Fig. 8.9a); Dr D. N. L. Ralphs (Fig. 4.1); Mr. H. Rogers, West Middlesex University Hospital, Isleworth (Fig. 10.12); Dr C. Rohrmann (Fig. 1.22); Dr P. Salmon London (Fig. 5.9); Dr D. E. Sharvill, St Saviour's Hospital, Hythe (Fig. 4.16); Professor F. E. Silverstein, University Hospital, Washington, and Professor G. N. J. Tytgat, Academic Medical Center, Amsterdam (Figs 1.5, 1.7–1.12, 1.17–1.19, 1.23, 1.24, 2.4, 2.5, 2.8, 2.9, 2.15, 2.16, 3.5, 3.8, 3.9, 3.12, 3.13, 3.15, 4.8, 4.9, 5.4, 6.2, 6.21–6.26, 8.1, 8.6a, 8.7a, 8.11, 8.14, 8.17, 8.18, 10.18, 10.20); Mr D. J. Spalton, St Thomas' Hospital, London (Fig. 9.25); Dr J. S. Tobias, University College Hospital, London, and Dr C. J. Williams, Southampton General Hospital, Southampton (Fig. 3.4); Professor J. D. Waye, Mt Sinai Hospital, New York, Professor J. E. Greenen, St Luke's Hospital, Racine, Wisconsin, Professor D. Fleischer, Georgetown University Hospital, Washington, and Professor R. P. Venu, Medical College of Wisconsin, Milwaukee (Figs 5.11, 10.19, 10.21, 10.22); Mr J. A. Williams (Fig. 6.30).

Contents

1. Gastro-oesophageal Reflux Disease

INTRODUCTION

Reflux of gastric contents into the lower oesophagus occurs in the majority of healthy individuals but is usually asymptomatic. Gastro-oesophageal reflux disease (GERD) occurs when the frequency and volume of this reflux is sufficient to generate symptoms. It is not necessarily accompanied by a hiatus hernia (this is found in up to 50% of the population) and rarely causes problems requiring medical advice. The vast sales of over-the-counter proprietary antacids indicate the high frequency of reflux symptoms and this is confirmed by general practice surveys (Fig. 1.1).

The factors responsible for the pathogenesis of GERD are shown in Fig. 1.2. The role of the various factors differs between patients but the advent of agents which virtually eliminate gastric acid production has demonstrated that acid and pepsin reflux into the lower oesophagus, possibly combined with impaired oesophageal peristaltic clearance, are the two dominant aetiological factors.

DIAGNOSIS

Symptoms

- Heartburn
- Chest pain
- Waterbrash
- Dysphagia
- Odynophagia

Heartburn and Chest Pain

These are the most common symptoms of GERD. Classically, retrosternal burning occurs about an hour after a meal, usually in the evening. They are precipitated or exacerbated by lying flat and stooping. Rapid relief by antacids is helpful diagnostically.

The differentiation of heartburn from angina, particularly where precordial pain also occurs, can be

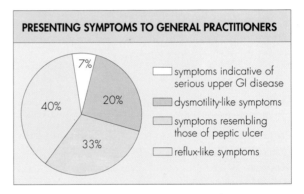

Fig. 1.1 Pie chart of presenting symptoms of upper gastrointestinal disease to GPs.

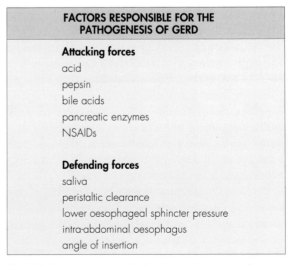

Fig. 1.2 Factors responsible for the pathogenesis of GERD.

very difficult. It is not unusual for oesophageal pain to radiate into the throat or jaw or radiate through to the back or into the arms. It may even be precipitated by exertion or emotional stress and be accompanied by minor ECG changes.

Waterbrash

Free reflux or regurgitation of gastric contents into the mouth produces a bitter burning taste, waterbrash, and may even lead to nocturnal coughing, wheezing or the finding of regurgitated gastric material on the pillow. Reflux-induced asthma is not usually due to aspiration but is attributed to the presence of refluxed gastric contents in the lower oesophagus causing diffuse bronchoconstriction mediated by pain receptors in the lower oesophagus.

Dysphagia and Odynophagia

Chronic reflux may induce scarring of the lower oesophagus, usually at the level of the oesophago-gastric junction, where stricture formation may eventually occur. Dysphagia may precede stricture formation by some years. It is often found in lower oesophageal inflammation but occasionally occurs in patients with motor abnormalities of the oesophagus. Pain on swallowing (odynophagia), particularly hot and cold liquids, also indicates severe oesophagitis.

MANAGEMENT

A careful history should elicit factors which may enable the patient to improve his symptoms without recourse to prescribed medications. These factors may include avoidance of a variety of drugs (Fig. 1.3) and/or dietary factors (Fig. 1.4).

Obesity significantly impairs the function of the lower oesophageal sphincter. Patients must understand the need to lose weight and avoid pathological eating habits. These include grazing after the early evening meal and taking unnecessary bedtime snacks. Avoidance of dietary factors known to promote reflux (see Fig. 1.4) is important, particularly in those who consume large amounts of coffee, citrus

---

DRUGS WHICH EXACERBATE GERD
Directly damaging to the mucosa
NSAIDs
edrophonium bromide
tetracyclines
slow-release potassium preparations
Causing relaxation of the lower oesophageal sphincter
anticholinergics
antidepressants
theophyllines
nitrates

Fig. 1.3 Drugs which exacerbate GERD.

DIETARY FACTORS WHICH PROMOTE REFLUX
citrus fruits
fruit juices
coffee
chocolate

Fig. 1.4 Dietary factors which promote reflux. These should be avoided by patients with GERD.

---

fruits or fruit juices. There is no doubt that smoking reduces lower oesophageal sphincter (LES) pressure and continuing tobacco consumption may mitigate virtually all therapeutic manipulations.

Controlled trials have shown the benefit of propping up the bedhead by at least the width of a house-brick and this is recommended for all patients whose symptoms are precipitated by lying flat. Sleeping propped up on several pillows is not sufficient.

Approximately 70% of patients respond to these non-pharmacological interventions. However, if no improvement occurs, further investigations are required before commencing pharmacological treatment.

INVESTIGATIONS

Patients with persistent symptoms of reflux disease, for whom long-term pharmacological therapy is being considered, should have the diagnosis con-

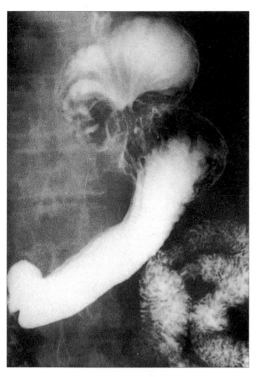

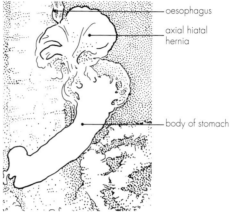

Fig. 1.5 Barium oesophagram demonstrating a large axial hiatus hernia. The proximal stomach has herniated through the diaphragm into the thorax.

oesophagus

axial hiatal hernia

body of stomach

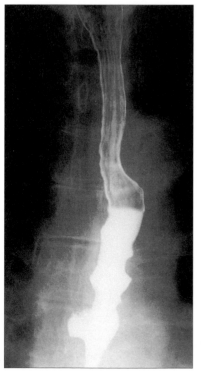

Fig. 1.6 Barium oesophagram showing characteristic nut-cracker oesophagus.

firmed. In these circumstances, a double contrast barium swallow and gastroscopy should be considered complementary. Undoubtedly, X-rays of the oesophagus with prone, head-down views provide excellent information on oesophageal function, particularly the size of a hiatus hernia and the degree of reflux (Fig. 1.5). Important additional views of oesophageal peristaltic function may also be obtained, but not if hyoscine bromide is routinely administered. In patients with chest pain, the finding of tertiary contractions with characteristic appearances of the nut-cracker oesophagus (Fig. 1.6) are extremely helpful.

Unfortunately, barium investigations have difficulty in accurately assessing the degree of inflammation at the lower end of the oesophagus, although they are much more accurate than endoscopy in determining the length of an oesophageal stricture.

Endoscopy may allow diagnosis of severe oesophageal inflammation in the presence of an apparently normal barium swallow, and it also

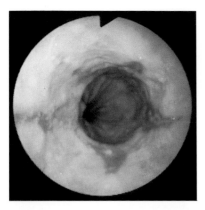

Fig. 1.7 Stage I reflux oesophagitis. Here, the reflux is quite extensive, with several linear, non-confluent red streaks extending up the oesophagus.

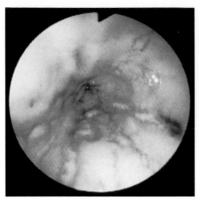

Fig. 1.8 Stage II reflux oesophagitis. White-based erosions extend up the oesophagus. Confluence but non-involvement of the entire circumference is noted.

Fig. 1.9 Stage III reflux oesophagitis. Denudation and friability are observed.

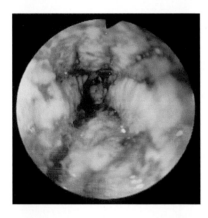

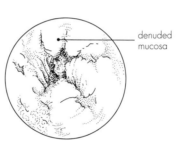

denuded mucosa

Fig. 1.10 Stage IVa reflux oesophagitis. The tight oesophageal stricture has associated ulceration and pseudodiverticula formation.

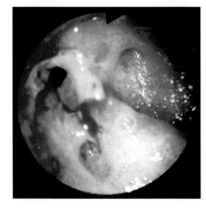

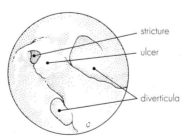

stricture

ulcer

diverticula

allows mucosal biopsy to be performed (Figs 1.7, 1.8, 1.9 and 1.10). In difficult cases where rarer causes of oesophageal symptoms may be responsible, such as viral oesophagitis or monilia, endoscopy is often the only way of making a firm diagnosis.

All patients with dysphagia should, where possible, have a barium swallow before endoscopy to exclude the rare occurrence of a pharyngeal pouch or of a high stricture, both of which may lead to perforation if blind endoscopy is performed (Figs 1.11 and 1.12). Where a barium swallow has shown that there is no stricturing and no evidence of possible oesophageal malignancy, empirical treatment with antacids or antagonists is perfectly appropriate; endoscopy will add very little further information.

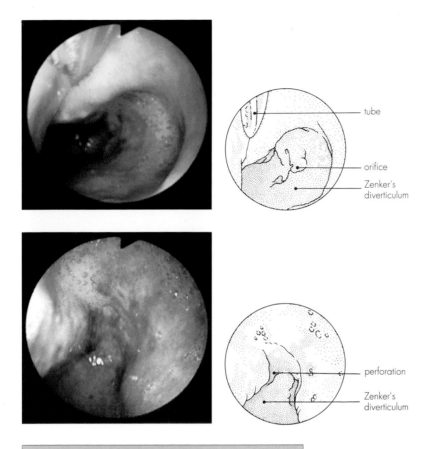

Fig. 1.11 Zenker's diverticulum. A tube has been passed into the oesophagus. The orifice into the oesophagus is difficult to see.

— tube

— orifice

— Zenker's diverticulum

Fig. 1.12 Zenker's diverticulum. The small perforation resulted from blind intubation.

— perforation

— Zenker's diverticulum

SPECIALIST INVESTIGATIONS
Oesophageal function tests
Bernstein test
edrophonium provocation
Oesophageal manometry
balloon distention
radionuclide transit
24–hour ambulatory pH monitoring

Fig. 1.13 Specialist investigations.

In patients who respond poorly to such an approach, endoscopy is mandatory. Quite often in these circumstances much more dramatic oesophageal inflammation is present than is expected by the findings, either on the history or on the patient's barium. General practitioners have to make their own decisions about which is the most appropriate investigation for patients with chronic reflux symptoms according to local availability. The costs of barium investigations and endoscopy are roughly equivalent. As a 'one-off', investigation endoscopy undoubtedly provides more information in the standard case.

SPECIALIST INVESTIGATIONS

In a minority of patients (usually those with intractable symptoms or atypical chest pain), where exercise tests and other studies of cardiac function are normal, more specialized oesophageal function tests (Fig. 1.13) may be necessary to confirm a diagnosis of reflux-induced oesophagospasm. These include 24-hour ambulatory pH monitoring (Fig. 1.14), in which a pH probe is inserted 5 cm above the gastro-oesophageal junction and a continuous recording is made for 24 hours and subsequently analysed by computer. Various definitions have been applied to findings so that an objective assessment of reflux can

1.5

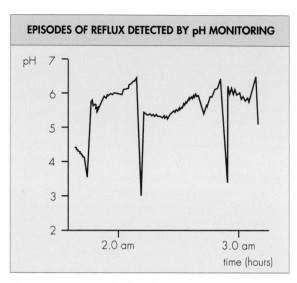

Fig. 1.14 Episodes of reflux detected by pH monitoring. Three periods of reflux with a pH less than 4 are shown.

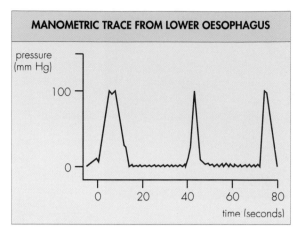

Fig. 1.15 Manometric trace from the lower oesophagus showing normal contractions on swallowing.

be compared between different laboratories. In general, the period of time for which the probe records a pH of less than 4 is taken to indicate the degree of reflux.

Unfortunately, more recent studies have shown an enormous variability between and within individuals with successive measurements. Even in normal subjects significant reflux often appears to occur without symptoms.

In patients in whom chest pain is thought to be related to contraction abnormalities of the oesophagus, oesophageal manometry may be helpful (Fig. 1.15). This should be confined to specialist centres with experience of the technique, which again is not wholly repeatable.

Other techniques to provoke chest pain by inducing oesophagospasm, include balloon distention of the oesophagus and edrophonium-induced contraction. All these tests should only be carried out in specialist units, and will be required for a very small minority of patients with reflux disease.

TREATMENT

It is necessary to take a detailed drug history from all patients and to replace, where possible, all agents which exacerbate GERD (see Fig. 1.3). Once pharmacological management is thought necessary, a diagnosis of the severity of the oesophagitis must be made, and here endoscopy is essential. Where oesophagitis is revealed, the various agents available should be considered. The aims of treatment must be clearly established: that is, relief of symptoms, prevention of stricturing and healing of ulceration.

Medical

Antacids

Although antacids rapidly relieve the symptoms of reflux in most cases, there is no evidence that these agents are effective in healing the inflamed oesophagus. Claims for greater efficacy for antacid combinations with alginates (which may increase lower oesophageal sphincter pressure), or with dimethicone (which forms a raft on the surface of the gastric contents), have not been proven in prospective, endoscopically controlled trials. Combinations of alginates with H_2-receptor antagonists have theoretical advantages which have still not been borne out by randomized trials. Antacid carbenoxolone combinations are of some benefit, but the salt- and water-retaining properties of carbenoxolone tend to contraindicate its usage, particularly in the elderly.

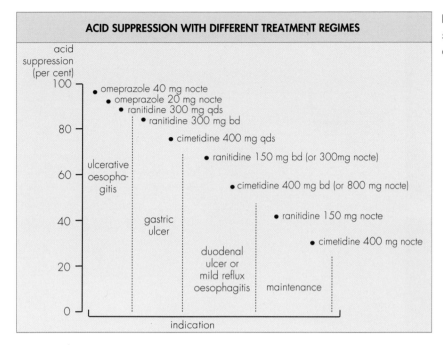

ACID SUPPRESSION WITH DIFFERENT TREATMENT REGIMES

acid suppression (per cent)

- omeprazole 40 mg nocte
- omeprazole 20 mg nocte
- ranitidine 300 mg qds
- ranitidine 300 mg bd
- cimetidine 400 mg qds
- ranitidine 150 mg bd (or 300mg nocte)
- cimetidine 400 mg bd (or 800 mg nocte)
- ranitidine 150 mg nocte
- cimetidine 400 mg nocte

ulcerative oesopha-gitis

gastric ulcer

duodenal ulcer or mild reflux oesophagitis

maintenance

indication

Fig. 1.16 Degree of acid suppression produced by different treatment regimes.

H₂-Receptor Antagonists

Suppression of gastric acid and pepsin production by H_2-receptor antagonists, such as cimetidine and ranitidine, is of proven value in healing reflux oesophagitis. In general, larger doses are needed than those used to heal duodenal ulcers. The efficacy of H_2-receptor antagonists in these circumstances is directly related to the degree of acid suppression achieved (Fig. 1.16). Full-dose maintenance therapy is usually required to prevent relapse in severe oesophagitis, but in milder cases a single nocturnal dose is usually sufficient providing patients comply with dietary restrictions and avoid precipitating factors.

Proton Pump Inhibition

Omeprazole, a substituted benzimidazole, inhibits the action of the proton pump on the gastric parietal cell, which pushes acid into the stomach lumen. It is a more powerful acid-suppressing agent than the H_2-receptor antagonists and has proved of great benefit in a high proportion of patients with apparently intractable oesophagitis. Controlled trials have shown much higher rates of healing of ulcerative oesophagitis than with either cimetidine or ranitidine (albeit in lower doses than would achieve equivalent acid suppression). Currently, omeprazole is only licensed for use in short, eight-week courses and is not advised for maintenance until its long-term safety is established.

Sucralfate

This complex of sulphated sucrose and aluminium hydroxide adheres directly to damaged mucosa. Patients often find the large tablets difficult to chew but they can be dissolved in water and a suspension of sucralfate is also available. Healing of resistant oesophagitis may be obtained but symptom relief is not as rapid as with the acid-suppressant agents.

Drugs Affecting Oesophageal Motility

Most reflux episodes are caused by inappropriate relaxation of the LES and therefore drugs which increase LES tone are usually not very successful in relieving symptoms. Nevertheless, dopamine antagonists, such as metoclopramide and domperidone, have been used in patients with oesophagitis but there is very little objective data to show that these drugs produce symptom relief or endoscopically observed healing. More promising may be cisapride, which works by releasing acetylcholine at nerve endings within the myenteric plexus. Apart from increasing motility throughout the gastrointestinal tract, cisapride increases the LES pressure and increases clearance of the contents of the lower

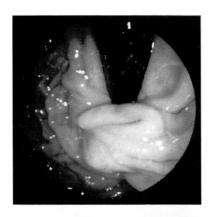

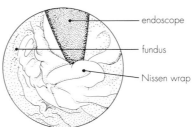

Fig. 1.17 The Nissen fundoplication. This is the operation of choice for patients with chronic reflux.

endoscope

fundus

Nissen wrap

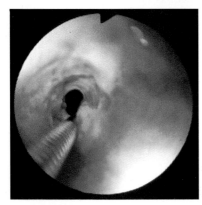

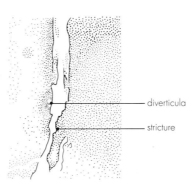

Fig. 1.18 Barium swallow showing a short stricture with a small mid-oesophageal diverticulum above.

diverticula

stricture

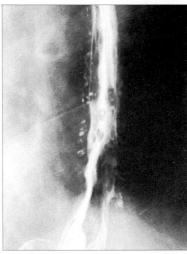

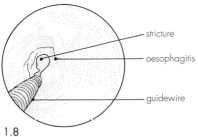

Fig. 1.19 Tight oesophageal stricture caused by reflux. A guidewire has been passed, under endoscopic guidance, to direct dilators and reduce the likelihood of a perforation during dilatation.

stricture

oesophagitis

guidewire

oesophagus by stimulating peristalsis. Controlled trials have shown cisapride to be of benefit in healing oesophagitis, although symptom relief is not obtained as quickly as with either H_2-receptor antagonists or omeprazole. Further studies on the combination of cisapride with acid suppressants are awaited.

Surgery

The proportion of patients with reflux disease who require surgery to control their symptoms is very small, particularly with the advent of proton pump inhibitors. Surgery is required where full medical treatment, combined with adherence to dietary advice, fails to control symptoms or in those patients with a long peptic stricture which is resistant to endoscopic dilatation.

Oesophageal function tests generally reveal that this group of patients are what may be described as

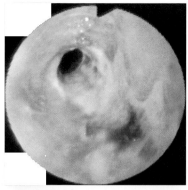

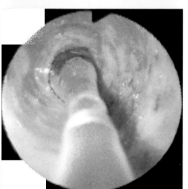

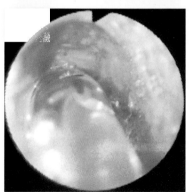

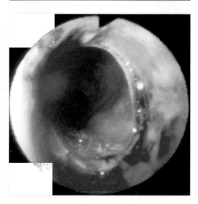

Fig. 1.20 Tight oesophageal stricture caused by reflux (left). Dilatation by the passage of mercury-filled bougies would be difficult, so a balloon-tipped catheter has been passed into the stricture under endoscopic guidance. The balloon is inflated to stretch the stricture. Finally, inspection of the stricture after dilatation shows that the lumen is open (extreme lower). The minimal bleeding was caused by the dilatation.

upright refluxers, that is, those patients in whom free reflux of gastric contents into the oesophagus occurs even when standing erect. This is mainly a mechanical problem which can only be alleviated by surgery. The most well-established, successful operation is the Nissen fundoplication (Fig. 1.17). This should ideally be performed by an experienced surgeon who carries out several operations of this nature per year. There are a variety of alternatives but, in the hands of an experienced surgeon, the fundoplication is undoubtedly the operation of choice for patients with chronic reflux symptoms.

COMPLICATIONS

Oesophageal Strictures

These are becoming less common but still occur in about 10% of patients with long-standing reflux. Presenting symptoms include dysphagia, usually for solids, and occasionally food bolus obstruction.

A barium swallow is necessary to delineate the site and length of the stricture and is of particular value when symptoms are long-standing and an oesophageal diverticulum is present (Fig. 1.18).

Medical treatment is usually ineffective. Endoscopy, biospy and dilatation maybe performed under mild sedation (Figs 1.19. and 1.20).

The use of proper doses of acid-supressant medication in patients with long-standing symptoms should prevent stricture formation. Once a stricture has formed, repeated dilatations may be necessary, with the risk of perforation always present (Fig. 1.21).

Oesophageal Ulcers

Reflux-associated oesophageal ulcers (Fig. 1.22) are rare and are often due to associated infections in debilitated patients or to NSAID therapy. They may also occur in association with Barrett's metaplasia.

Barrett's Metaplasia

This is most likely to occur in patients with severe, continuous reflux. Normal squamous mucosa is

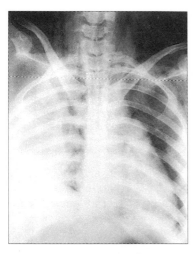

Fig. 1.21 Radiograph showing consequences of oesophageal perforation following dilatation of an oesophageal stricture. There is a large right, pleural effusion, mediastinal emphysema and gross surgical emphysema in the neck and upper chest wall.

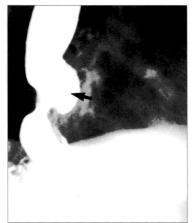
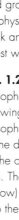

Fig. 1.22 Barium oesophagram showing a large oesophageal ulcer in the distal third of the oesophagus. The ulcer (arrow) extends into the tissue adjacent to the oesophagus.

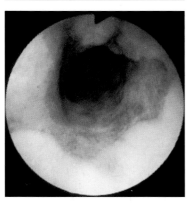

Fig. 1.23 Barrett's metaplasia. The squamocolumnar junction has moved proximally in the oesophagus. It is distinct but irregular, with islands of columnar mucosa.

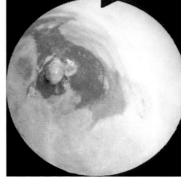

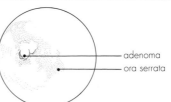

adenoma
ora serrata

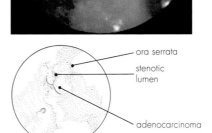

ora serrata
stenotic lumen
adenocarcinoma

Fig. 1.24 Upper: oesophageal adenoma in a patient with Barrett's metaplasia. Due to underlying medical problems, this was removed endoscopically using a polypectomy technique. Lower: two years later, an adenocarcinoma is found in the same area. The tumour was superficial but had metastasized.

replaced by columnar epithelium that is congenital in origin or results from desquamation of a chronically inflamed mucosa. As the replacement occurs, the squamocolumnar junction migrates caudally (Fig. 1.23). Barrett's metaplasia is undoubtedly premalignant and requires long-term endoscopic surveillance (Fig. 1.24).

POINTS TO REMEMBER

- Ensure compliance with advice on diet, stopping smoking and weight reduction before offering pharmacological agents
- Use adequate doses of acid-suppressant medication for healing and maintenance
- Dysphagia always requires investigation
- Fit patients with intractable disease should be offered surgery

2. Peptic Ulcer

INTRODUCTION

Epidemiology

Peptic ulcer will affect up to 10% of the population at some time. The disease is commoner in men than women. Accurate data on the incidence and prevalence of the disease are limited; however, there is no doubt that there has been a steady and significant fall in the occurrence of perforated peptic ulcer since 1950. This decline is mainly concentrated in younger subjects, with no apparent change in the rates of perforation or mortality in the elderly.

According to death certification in the UK, approximately 5,000 deaths per year are attributed to peptic ulcer, but autopsy studies on subjects who die suddenly at home indicate that this figure may be a serious underestimate. Most peptic ulcers are probably asymptomatic or associated with symptoms which are mild and indistinguishable from other less serious causes of dyspepsia. Interval endoscopies have revealed silent ulcers in up to 40% of asymptomatic patients taking part in maintenance studies of peptic ulcer healing.

These factors have a major influence on the management of peptic ulcer, where the therapeutic problems tend to be concentrated on prevention of relapse rather than acute healing.

Pathogenesis

The traditional see-saw model indicates that peptic ulcers arise from an imbalance between acid/pepsin secretion and mucosal resistance. Only 30% of peptic ulcer patients secrete increased amounts of acid, and peptic ulcers generally develop when there is disruption of the mucosal response to injury. Among the known major factors which impair mucosal resistance are the use of non-steroidal anti-inflammatory drugs (NSAIDs) and *Helicobacter pylori* infection. Fig. 2.1 summarizes the pathogenesis of peptic ulceration.

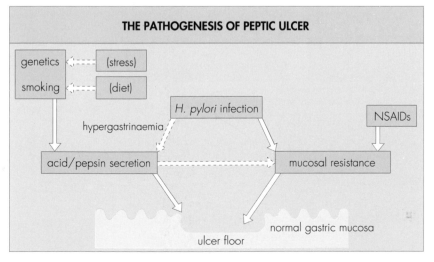

Fig. 2.1 The pathogenesis of peptic ulcer.

Genetics

Duodenal ulcer is more common in subjects with blood group O then in those with A, B or AB. The blood group association is most marked with complicated peptic ulcer.

Hyperpepsinogenaemia is inherited as an autosomal dominant characteristic and is associated with an increased tendency to duodenal ulcers. These genetic factors interact with external environmental influences (such as smoking) to promote the formation of peptic ulcers in an undetermined proportion of peptic ulcer patients.

Smoking

There is an undoubted association between cigarette smoking and peptic ulceration. Smoking delays the

---

SMOKING AND PEPTIC ULCER

increased acid secretory capacity
decreased mucosal blood flow
decreased prostaglandin production

Fig. 2.2 The pathogenesis of smoking and peptic ulcer.

healing of ulcers and increases the rate of relapse. Smokers are more likely to require surgery, as the response to standard healing agents is impaired, and are also more likely to suffer complications after surgery and die as a result of the disease. Possible mechanisms to explain the detrimental effect of smoking are shown in Fig. 2.2.

Diet

There is no current evidence to support the idea of any single dietary factor or combination of factors being clearly related to an increased risk of duodenal ulceration. Careful surveys have revealed that peptic ulcer patients do not seem to have a greater intake of spicy foods, caffeine or alcohol than healthy subjects. Also, it seems that milk appears to increase gastric acid production. There are some data to suggest that peptic ulcer patients take their beverages at much higher temperatures than non-ulcer subjects, but the relationship between this curious finding and the pathogenesis of peptic ulceration is unclear.

Stress

Scattered case reports and occasional controlled studies suggest an association between psycho-social

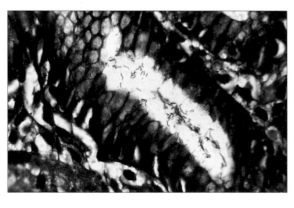

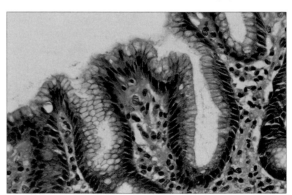

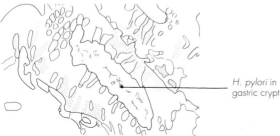
H. pylori in gastric crypt

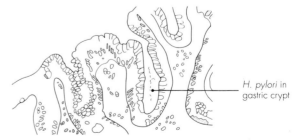
H. pylori in gastric crypt

Fig. 2.3 Histological appearances of H. pylori infection.

stresses and peptic ulcer. However, the difficulty in quantifying stress for an individual, and the inability, at present, to reproduce measurements of the gastric or duodenal response to stress, has inhibited the establishment of any clear relationship between stress and peptic ulcer.

Helicobacter pylori *and Peptic Ulcer*

Helicobacter pylori has been found in all human population studies, increasing in frequency with advancing age. In the West, at least 50% of those over the age of 50 are infected. By contrast, a greater proportion of Third World subjects are infected in childhood. The source of infection is unknown, although, in the West, the carrying rate among abattoir workers who handle carcasses is higher than that of their office-based control colleagues. There are isolated reports of infection in baboons and ferrets, but human to human spread is the most likely form of transmission.

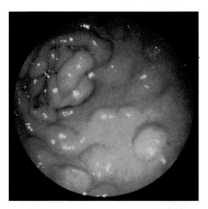

Fig. 2.4 Gastric metaplasia of the duodenal bulb.

H. pylori has been found in the gastric antrum (Fig. 2.3) of 90 to 95% of patients with duodenal ulcer and 75% of patients with gastric ulcer. Approximately 50% of patients with ulcer-negative dyspepsia are infected, as are at least 20% of the healthy population. These very high rates of infection raise the question of whether *H. pylori* is a significant factor in the aetiology of peptic ulcer or merely an innocent (and diverting) bystander.

POSSIBLE PATHOGENIC MECHANISMS OF *H. PYLORI*

If *H. pylori* is damaging to the gastro-duodenal mucosa this may either be by direct means, such as local toxin release, or by indirect means, i.e. by generating an inappropriate rise in acid pepsin secretion.

The curious and unique ability of its urease enzyme to generate local alkaline conditions, by the splitting of urease to ammonia, appears to result in an inappropriate hypergastrinaemia. Eradication of the organism results in a fall in basal and stimulated gastrin secretion. This very neat explanation for the role of *H. pylori* in the pathogenesis of peptic ulceration has been tested in very small numbers of patients to date, but is supported by the experimental data.

Direct colonization of areas of gastric metaplasia in the duodenal bulb is another possible pathogenic mechanism (Fig. 2.4). Abnormal acid secretion may induce gastric metaplasia in the duodenal cap allowing *H. pylori* to migrate into the duodenum where it may initiate duodenitis and subsequently duodenal ulceration (Fig. 2.5).

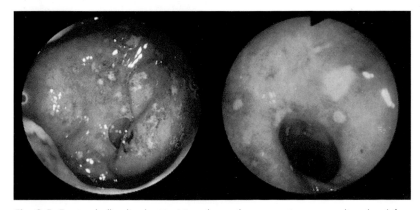
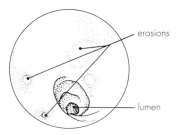

Fig. 2.5 Erosive bulboduodenitis. Note the erythematous ring surrounding the defects.

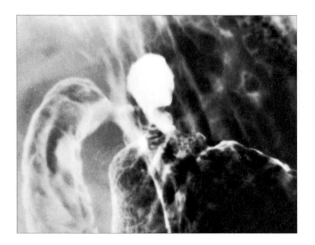

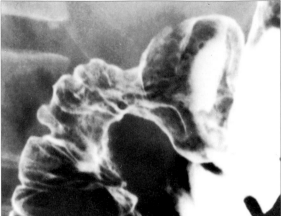

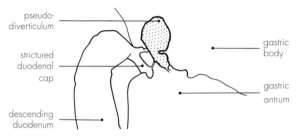

pseudo-
diverticulum

gastric
body

strictured
duodenal
cap

gastric
antrum

descending
duodenum

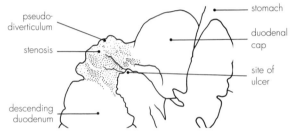

pseudo-
diverticulum

stomach

stenosis

duodenal
cap

site of
ulcer

descending
duodenum

Fig. 2.6 Barium meal showing gross deformity of the duodenal cap with stricturing and pseudodiverticula formation, making it difficult to detect a central ulcer crater.

Fig. 2.7 Hypotonic duodenogram of a post-bulbar ulcer. The ulcer itself is difficult to see although the deformity with stenosis and some pseudodiverticular change is evident.

A key factor in understanding these problems is knowing the means by which *H. pylori* becomes adherent to gastric mucosal cells and glands. Recent work indicates that the urease enzyme protects the organism from acid digestion.

If *H. pylori* is of pathogenic significance, the low 'hit' rate amongst chronic carriers and the major regional differences in the distribution of peptic ulcer must be explained. Perhaps the single most important factor supporting the role of *H. pylori* in peptic ulcers is the dramatic reduction in the relapse rate if *H. pylori* is eradicated.

For some years it has been suggested that Bismuth salts may heal duodenal ulcers which then tend to relapse less often than those healed by H_2-receptor antagonists. The most recent studies indicate that apparently the key factor determining relapse is the presence or absence of *H. pylori*, which is sensitive to Bismuth.

However, some of these studies can be criticized for inadequate blinding, small numbers, low initial overall healing and problems with sampling. Ulcers recur in patients without *H. pylori* infection and, in some studies, the rates of ulcer recurrence are unaffected by the presence or absence of the organism.

At present, then, there is not enough evidence to promote *H. pylori* eradication as the primary aim of peptic ulcer treatment. Even so, attempts to eradicate the organism may be justified in patients with refractory ulcers and those who frequently relapse.

DIAGNOSIS

Symptoms

- Epigastric pain – often nocturnal, relieved by antacids or H_2-receptor antagonists, and relieved by food
- Vomiting
- Weight loss

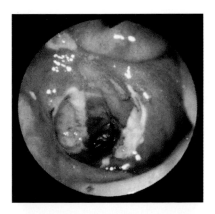

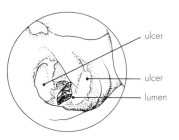

Fig. 2.8 Kissing ulcers in the bulb are found on opposite walls at the same site.

ulcer

ulcer

lumen

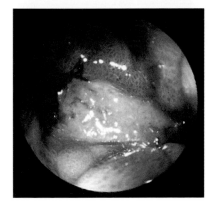

Fig. 2.9 Large duodenal ulcer of the posterior wall with marked erythema and friability of the border.

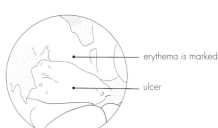

erythema is marked

ulcer

The clinical diagnosis of peptic ulceration is often very difficult. Computer analysis of the symptoms related to the presence of an ulcer suggest that those listed above are most helpful. A drug history is clearly of great importance, giving particular attention to NSAIDs and over the counter analgesics.

Epigastric pain may or may not be related temporarily to meals. Characteristically, the pain is recurrent and longstanding, often nocturnal, and may be relieved by vomiting. Guarding may be present and, in complicated cases, signs of recent haemorrhage or chronic anaemia may be helpful. Certainly, in elderly patients, the first presentation of a peptic ulcer may be a massive haemorrhage or fatal perforation. Common associated symptoms which often confuse the clinician include flatulence, heartburn and bloating after meals. Visible peristalsis, upper abdominal distention, and a succussion splash may indicate the presence of pyloric stenosis. Duodenal and gastric ulcers cannot be differentiated clinically.

Diagnosis

Peptic ulcers may be diagnosed either by double contrast barium meal examination or upper gastrointestinal endoscopy (see Figs 2.6, 2.7, 2.8 and 2.9). The various advantages and disadvantages of the techniques have been discussed at great length over recent years. The local availability of services is probably the main determining factor, particularly where family practitioners have open access to radiological departments. However, the benefits endoscopy can provide, with the ability to biopsy the mucosa in the peripyloric area to exclude or confirm the presence of *H. pylori*, may lead in future to a greater demand for endoscopy as the first line of investigation. This will produce obvious logistical problems for hospital-based gastrointestinal units and it may be that some endoscopic services will, in the future, be community based.

Gastric Ulcer

Gastric ulcers (Figs 2.10 and 2.11) always require biopsy and repeat endoscopy six to eight weeks after the start of treatment. If the ulcer does not heal repeat biopsy should be performed and endoscopy again arranged until complete healing is achieved.

INVESTIGATION

Which Patients Require Investigation?

The huge increase in demand for the diagnosis and treatment of dyspepsia is presumably led by the belief that a significant proportion of patients presenting with upper gastrointestinal symptoms have serious organic disease. Prospective surveys which attempt to link symptoms to the results of investigations help to identify subsets of patients in whom endoscopy or a barium meal is clearly indicated, and those with whom blind therapy is reasonable (see Fig. 2.12).

Younger patients with a strong family history of peptic ulcer should be offered investigation. Difficulties arise, however, in younger subjects with recurrent symptoms, which reappear as soon as medication is withdrawn. Here investigation may be seen as a cheaper alternative to long-term treatment with expensive and possibly unnecessary therapies.

TREATMENT

The aims of treatment are threefold: first, relief of the patient's symptoms; second, healing of the ulcer; and, third, prevention of relapse (known to be up to 70% in the first year of healing for duodenal ulcer and 95 to 100% for gastric ulcer). The various therapeutic options are shown in Fig. 2.13.

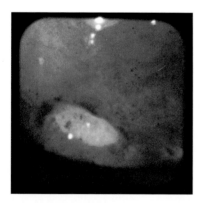
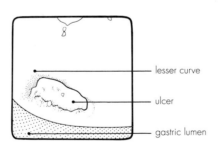

Fig. 2.10 Endoscopic view of a chronic lesser curve gastric ulcer.

lesser curve

ulcer

gastric lumen

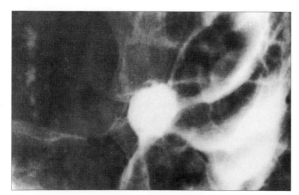
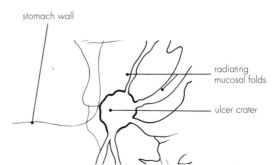

stomach wall

radiating mucosal folds

ulcer crater

Fig. 2.11 Barium meal showing a large, benign, lesser curve gastric ulcer with gastric folds radiating from the edge of the ulcer crater.

INDICATIONS FOR INVESTIGATION

age >45 years
previous history of peptic ulcer
use of NSAIDs/aspirin
weight loss
nocturnal pain relieved by antacids
vomiting

Fig. 2.12 Indications for investigation of peptic ulcer.

THERAPEUTIC OPTIONS IN THE TREATMENT OF PEPTIC ULCER

Adverse factors that need to be reduced
smoking
NSAIDs
(alcohol)
poor eating pattern

Drug treatment
antacids
H_2-receptor antagonists
anticholinergics
tripotassium dicitratobismuthate
sucralfate
liquorice extract
prostaglandins
substitute benzimidazoles

Fig. 2.13 Therapeutic options in the treatment of peptic ulcer.

ADVERSE EFFECTS OF CIMETIDINE

diarrhoea
confusion in the very ill or elderly
antiandrogen effects
interfere with the metabolism of
    warfarin
    diazepam
    propranolol
    phenytoin
    theophylline
    chlormethiazole

Fig. 2.14 Adverse effects of cimetidine.

Acute Healing

In practice, although all the treatments shown in Fig. 2.13 eventually heal ulcers, the safest and best evaluated are the histamine H_2-receptor antagonists. The ability of this group of drugs to reduce the volume and concentration of gastric acid and pepsin secretion results in 80 to 90% healing of duodenal ulcers and 70 to 80% healing of gastric ulcers after four- to twelve-week courses of treatment with once-daily doses. Side effects are minimal, with some theoretical disadvantage to cimetidine which may interfere with the metabolism of drugs which use the hepatic cyto-chrome P-450 system (see Fig. 2.14).

Dosage and Timing

Acute Treatment

Once-daily administration of 800 mg cimetidine or 300 mg ranitidine before bedtime will heal 80 to 90% of duodenal ulcers after four weeks. Larger doses given two or three times daily may be required to heal gastric ulcers. Similar rates of healing can be achieved with a once daily dose of nizatidine and famotidine. Symptoms are usually relieved within three to five weeks. A second course of H_2-receptor antagonists may be required to heal approximately 10% of resistant cases. At the end of eight weeks a small proportion (3 to 8%) of ulcers will remain unhealed.

Refractory Ulcers

Further endoscopy (and in gastric ulcers repeat biopsy to exclude malignancy) is necessary to confirm that the ulcer is still present. In patients with duodenal ulcer, biopsies should be taken from the antral mucosa, within 2 cm of the pylorus (see Figs 2.15 and 2.16), and should be cultured and examined histologically for the presence of *H. pylori*. The choice of treatment now lies between more powerful acid suppression (increased doses of H_2-receptor antagonists, omeprazole) or *H. pylori* eradication. As the H_2-receptor antagonists and omeprazole do not appear to alter the natural history of peptic ulcer at this stage, triple therapy (see Fig. 2.17) is indicated if

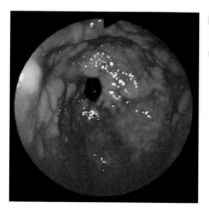

Fig.2.15 Antral intestinal metaplasia

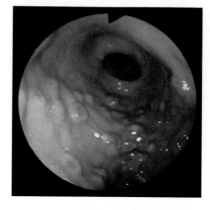

Fig. 2.16 Erosive antral gastritis.

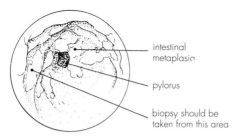

intestinal metaplasia

pylorus

biopsy should be taken from this area

TRIPLE THERAPY TO ELIMINATE *H. PYLORI*

Tripotassium dicitratobismuthate: one tablet four times a day for four weeks (half an hour before each of the main meals of the day and two hours after the evening meal). Avoid milk during the course of treatment.

In the last week of treatment administer

Metronidazole: 400 mg three times a day for five days.

Amoxycillin: 500 mg four times a day for five days.

Fig. 2.17 Triple therapy to eliminate *H. pylori*.

---

long-term maintenance treatment is not under consideration.

In elderly patients and in those who may be poorly compliant, short-term treatment with omeprazole and long-term maintenance with H_2-receptor antagonists may be a better option. In younger patients, triple therapy (see Fig. 2.17) should be offered with repeat endoscopy and antral biopsy at the end of treatment.

Nausea and diarrhoea are common side effects and this course of treatment should not be undertaken lightly. *H. pylori* eradication will be achieved in 70% of patients treated. Furthermore, duodenal ulcers healed in this manner have a 10 to 30% relapse rate after twelve months compared with up to 70% in patients treated with H_2-receptor antagonists.

Intermittent or Maintenance Treatment?

The failure of H_2-receptor antagonists to modify the natural history of peptic ulcers has led to consider-

able debate on the advice and treatment which should be given to patients whose ulcers relapse on stopping treatment. At one end of the spectrum is the view that peptic ulceration is analogous to hypertension – a disease that requires lifelong treatment. At the other end, prompt relapse is an indication of the need for definitive surgery. Fig. 2.18 indicates a reasonable approach to long-term management.

In practice, patients tend to prefer long-term treatment to the surgical alternatives, particularly when they are informed that maintenance treatment not only reduces the relapse rate but also the risks of long-term complications.

Other Approaches

Medical

Primary treatment with sucralfate, liquorice extract, prostaglandins and anticholinergics is less acceptable as these drugs do not provide rapid symptom relief

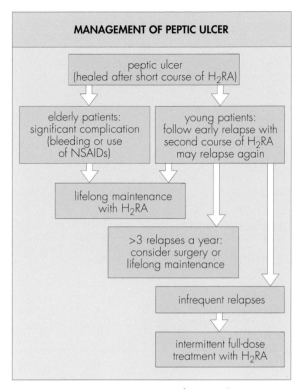

MANAGEMENT OF PEPTIC ULCER

peptic ulcer
(healed after short course of H$_2$RA)

elderly patients:
significant complication
(bleeding or use
of NSAIDs)

young patients:
follow early relapse with
second course of H$_2$RA
may relapse again

lifelong maintenance
with H$_2$RA

>3 relapses a year:
consider surgery or
lifelong maintenance

infrequent relapses

intermittent full-dose
treatment with H$_2$RA

Fig. 2.18 Long-term management of peptic ulcer.

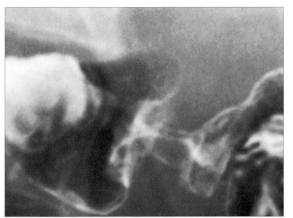

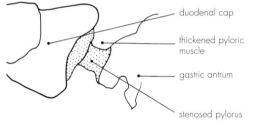

duodenal cap

thickened pyloric
muscle

gastric antrum

stenosed pylorus

Fig. 2.19 Barium meal showing pyloric stenosis due to hypertrophy of the pyloric muscle.

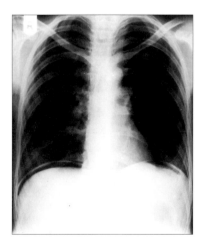

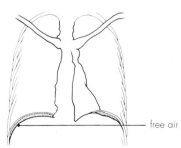

free air

Fig. 2.20 Radiograph showing free air under both diaphragms following perforation of a duodenal ulcer.

and may be poorly tolerated either due to side effects or lack of palatability.

Surgical

The efficacy of the H$_2$-receptor antagonists in the treatment of peptic ulcer has dramtically reduced the elective operation rates for peptic ulcer. Most surgeons will perform a handful of acid-reducing operations per year, the majority being carried out to treat complications of peptic ulceration (pyloric stenosis (Fig. 2.19), perforation (Fig. 2.20), haemorrhage (see Fig. 2.21)), rather than dealing with failures of medical

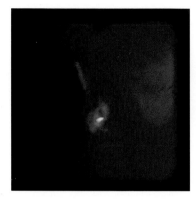

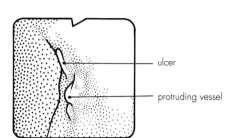

Fig. 2.21 Endoscopic view of an ulcer with a protruding vessel.

ulcer

protruding vessel

treatment. Highly selective vagotomy is an excellent acid reducing operation with few complications and good long-term results. However, the advent of highly potent acid suppressant medication (omeprazole) may render even this procedure, with its few indications, largely obsolete.

POINTS TO REMEMBER

Peptic ulcers which fail to heal

• Check compliance
• Stop the patient smoking
• Avoid NSAIDs and aspirin
• Ask for repeat endoscopy

3. Upper Gastrointestinal Cancer

OESOPHAGEAL CARCINOMA

Introduction

More than 90% of primary carcinomas of the oesophagus are of squamous-cell origin. Adenocarcinomas usually arise in the lower third of the oesophagus in metaplastic or dysplastic columnar-lined epithelium. Most oesophageal carcinomas present late, symptoms are distressing and curative treatment is not possible.

In China, an area of high prevalence, screening by oesophageal cytology allows the early identification of up to 70% of tumours. In western countries, with a much lower prevalence of oesophageal carcinoma, there is no consensus as to the value of screening even in those individuals known to have a higher risk for developing a tumour.

Epidemiology

There is an astonishing variation in the prevalence of this common malignancy. In the USA and Western Europe there is a prevalence of 5 to 7/100,000 per annum, with much higher rates in parts of Africa, and rising to as much as 184/100,000 per annum in women in parts of Iran (Fig. 3.1). In most countries it is commoner in men. The risk factors and diseases associated with oesophageal carcinoma are shown in Fig. 3.2

Pathogenesis

Approximately 90% of oesophageal carcinomas are of squamous-cell origin. The degree of histological differentiation varies widely but does not correlate with clinical presentation or outcome. Initial spread of the tumour is longitudinal or extramural, with

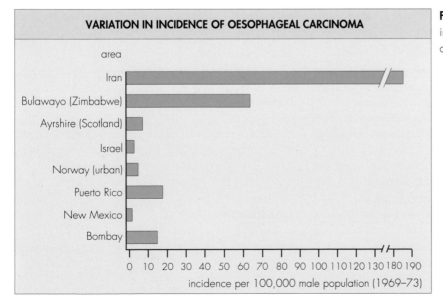

Fig. 3.1 Geographical incidence of oesophageal carcinoma.

RISK FACTORS AND DISEASES ASSOCIATED WITH OESOPHAGEAL CARCINOMA

Risk factors
smoking
alcohol ingestion
corrosive injury of the oesophagus

Diseases
achalasia of the oesophagus
iron deficiency with an oesophageal web
  (Plummer–Vinson or Paterson–Kelly–Brown syndrome)
tylosis (a rare genetic disorder with hyperkeratosis of
  palms and soles, and a 100% chance of oesophageal
  carcinoma)
other carcinomas of the head and neck

Fig. 3.2 Risk factors and diseases associated with oesophageal carcinoma.

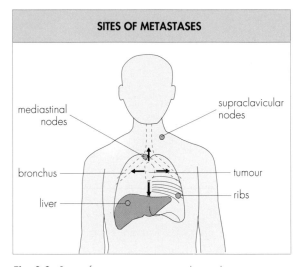

SITES OF METASTASES

mediastinal nodes
supraclavicular nodes
bronchus
tumour
liver
ribs

Fig. 3.3 Sites of metastases in oesophageal carcinoma.

early lymphatic spread. Most tumours are at least 4 cm in size at diagnosis and, if the tumour is greater than 5 cm in size, there is a 90% probability of regional lymph nodes being involved. Further spread is predominantly to the liver and lungs (Fig. 3.3), but bony metastases also occur. Approximately 5% of patients develop a fistula between the oesophagus and the trachea or a main bronchus.

A minority (less than 1% in Europe) of squamous-cell carcinomas of the oesophagus are confined to the mucosa and submucosa. These are usually an incidental finding during endoscopy for other reasons.

DIAGNOSIS

Symptoms

Oesophageal cancer
- Dysphagia
- Odynophagia (pain on swallowing)
- Anorexia and weight loss
- Anaemia
- Aching chest pain
- Cough and aspiration pneumonia
- Haematemesis
- Hypercalcaemia (rare)

Dysphagia is almost always the first symptom and, unfortunately, does not occur until there is extensive disease. Dysphagia must always be investigated. Some patients will indicate the apparent site of 'hold-up' when they are swallowing but this is a poor indication of the anatomical localization of any lesion. Dysphagia is typically 'progressive' with initial difficulty associated with meat or bread, followed by an ability to swallow only a semi-solid and eventually a liquid diet.

Odynophagia is due to infection, inflammation or obstruction of the oesophagus. It is a clear indicator of oesophageal disease and warrants early investigation. Odynophagia may occur with dysphagia.

The remaining symptoms indicate serious disease but are not specific to the oesophagus. Chest pain occurs late in the course of the disease and is due to metastatic spread of the tumour. A recurrent cough and episodes of pneumonia suggest a tracheo-oesophageal fistula.

Examination

Physical examination may reveal obvious weight loss, lymph node spread (especially cervical) or hepatomegaly due to hepatic metastases (see Fig. 3.3).

Investigation

There may be an iron deficiency anaemia, suggesting slow blood loss, and abnormal liver blood tests suggesting hepatic mestastases. Although uncommon, hypercalcaemia should be sought since treatment

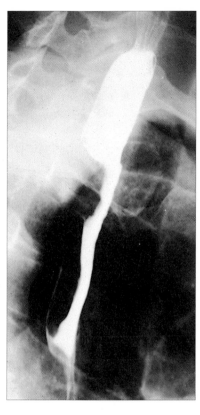

Fig. 3.4 Carcinoma of the upper oesophagus. The obvious constriction in the barium flow is typical of a carcinoma.

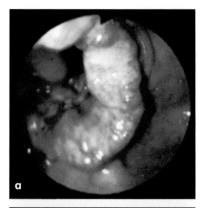

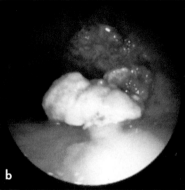

Fig. 3.5 a. This elevated squamous-cell carcinoma involves more than 75% of the oesophageal circumference. **b.** Typical squamous-cell carcinoma, with raised margins and a central ulcer.

will produce considerable symptomatic improvement. A chest X-ray may be normal or show mediastinal widening and occasionally bony metastases.

A barium swallow usually reveals a narrower oesophagus with irregular mucosa (Fig. 3.4). Benign strictures of the oesophagus are usually smooth and tapering whilst malignant strictures are asymmetric. In addition to identifying the probable nature of a stricture, a barium swallow usually allows examination of the hypopharynx, distal oesophagus and stomach. Endoscopy (Fig. 3.5) allows histological confirmation.

Most gastroenterologists will consider a barium swallow as the first line of investigation for dysphagia, whilst some will proceed directly to endoscopy.

Treatment

Surgery

Curative surgery may be attempted in the minority of patients who are reasonably well nourished and who show no evidence of metastatic disease, either clinic-

ally or by chest X-ray, upper abdominal ultrasound and/or CT scan. As laparoscopy is more sensitive than ultrasound, it is more effective in detecting hepatic metastases, although endoscopic ultrasound is being evaluated as a staging technique. Even when an apparently curative surgical procedure is performed there is high operative mortality and a 5-year survival rate of less than 10%. There is no evidence that combining surgery with pre- or post-operative radiotherapy improves survival.

Radiotherapy

Radiotherapy is of little value in adenocarcinomas of the distal oesophagus but is extensively used for the more common squamous-cell carcinomas. In many centres, patients who are elderly, or in whom curative surgery is not feasible, are offered palliative radiotherapy. This practice is based on the assumption that surgery is more likely to achieve a 'cure'; however, there is no evidence to support this. Unfortunately, accurate comparative trials of surgery or radiotherapy as primary treatment are not available. Radiotherapy avoids the early operative mortal-

OTHER MODES OF PALLIATIVE TREATMENT

Oesophageal dilatation
Eder-Puestow 'olives' over a guidewire
tapered dilators, e.g. Celestin
balloon dilators, e.g. Rigiflex

Oesophageal prosthesis
usually inserted endoscopically, e.g. Nottingham tube

Endoscopic tumour ablation
laser photocoagulation
absolute alcohol injection inducing tumour necrosis

Fig. 3.6 Other modes of palliative treatment.

AN OESOPHAGEAL PROSTHESIS

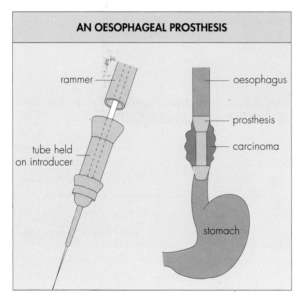

Fig. 3.7 An oesophageal prosthesis. The Nottingham tube is inserted after oesophageal dilatation. Careful positioning of the tube under fluoroscopic or endoscopic control is essential.

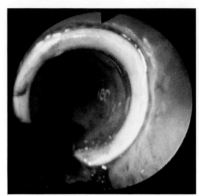

Fig. 3.8 An oesophageal prosthesis placed, under endoscopic guidance, through the narrowed area of the oesophagus affected by a deep, infiltrating squamous-cell carcinoma.

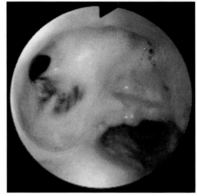

Fig. 3.9 Tracheo-oesophageal fistula, caused by an ulcerating oesophageal squamous-cell carcinoma. The fistula tract orifice is clearly seen.

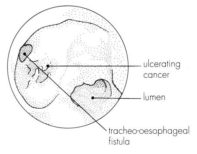

ity of a surgical approach but dysphagia may worsen during the first week or so of treatment. Radiation oesophagitis or infection, either viral or more commonly candidal, may occasionally occur.

Other Approaches

Effective chemotherapy regimes for treatment or palliation are not available. Even so, other modes of therapy are available (Fig. 3.6) and are all used to achieve or preserve sufficient patency of the oesophageal lumen to allow swallowing. The techniques used will depend both on individual patient needs and local expertise. Oesophageal dilatation is performed prior to the other procedures, and previous radiotherapy is not a contraindication. An oesophageal prosthesis (Fig. 3.7) is often used, espe-

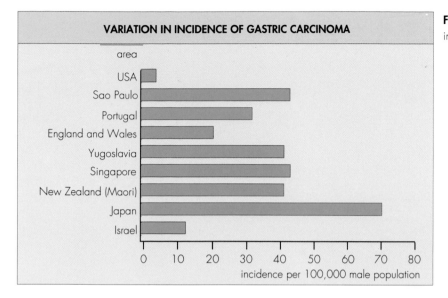

VARIATION IN INCIDENCE OF GASTRIC CARCINOMA

area

USA
Sao Paulo
Portugal
England and Wales
Yugoslavia
Singapore
New Zealand (Maori)
Japan
Israel

0 10 20 30 40 50 60 70 80

incidence per 100,000 male population

Fig. 3.10 Geographical incidence of gastric carcinoma.

POSSIBLE RISK FACTORS FOR GASTRIC CARCINOMA

age

socio-economic status

family history

diet (nitrites, salt)

previous partial gastrectomy

pernicious anaemia

intestinal metaplasia and chronic atrophic gastritis

Fig. 3.11 Possible risk factors for gastric carcinoma.

cially if there is perforation of a malignant stricture (Fig. 3.8) or if a tracheo-oesophageal fistula has developed (Fig. 3.9). Although very useful for some patients, an oesophageal prosthesis may become blocked, therefore patients have to be advised to eat small, frequent semi-solid or liquid meals in an upright position.

Prognosis

The outlook is appalling and has not changed over several decades, despite all the improvements in investigation and post-operative care. Less than 10% of patients will survive 5 years whatever the mode of treatment used. For the majority of patients, how-ever, effective palliation including maintenance of adequate nutrition can be provided.

POINTS TO REMEMBER

• Dysphagia and odynophagia must always be investigated
• Treatment is rarely curative
• Effective palliation is possible

GASTRIC CARCINOMA

Epidemiology

There is a large variation in the prevalence of gastric carcinoma, not only between countries but also between different areas of the same country. The highest prevalence is in Japan where there is an annual mortality rate of 70/100,000 compared with a figure of 6/100,000 in the USA (Fig. 3.10). The incidence is falling gradually in many countries. Gastric carcinoma has been linked to a high dietary intake of salt and high nitrite levels in drinking water, but there are conflicting studies which do not confirm this association. Other risk factors are shown in Fig. 3.11. There is continuing debate about the possible association of gastric cancer with previous partial gastrectomy, intestinal metaplasia and pernicious anaemia.

Pathogenesis

Gastric carcinoma is classified as early gastric cancer (EGC; Fig. 3.12) and advanced gastric cancer (AGC; Fig. 3.13). The distinction between the two is histological, and based entirely on disease limited to the mucosa and submucosa. EGC may still be present despite local lymph node involvement. EGC was first described in Japan. It accounts for up to 5% of cases in western countries. Unfortunately, most patients present with advanced disease.

DIAGNOSIS

Symptoms and signs

Early gastric cancer
- usually asymptomatic
- occasional anaemia

Advanced gastric cancer
- weight loss
- anorexia
- epigastric pain
- vomiting
- epigastric mass
- hepatomegaly
- ascites
- lymphadenopathy

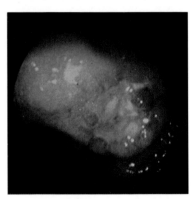

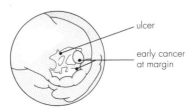

Fig. 3.12 Early gastric cancer. Gastric ulceration and early cancer at the margin are evident.

ulcer

early cancer at margin

Early Gastric Cancer

There are usually no symptoms and the results of physical examination are normal. A minority of patients with EGC complain of nausea or epigastric discomfort and fullness.

Advanced Gastric Cancer

The typical symptoms of AGC are those of weight loss and upper abdominal pain. Vomiting is more likely when the tumour encroaches on the pylorus, obstructing the passage of gastric contents. Tumours arising within the fundus or cardia of the stomach frequently invade the lower oesophagus and the patient may present with dysphagia. If there are abnormal physical signs these suggest extensive disease.

Investigations

Many gastroenterologists encourage immediate referral of patients over the age of 50, who are presenting with epigastric pain for the first time, for endoscopy or barium meal examination. The hope is that this policy will greatly facilitate the identification of patients who have EGC.

The diagnosis of AGC is usually straightforward. A barium meal may reveal a typical proliferative gastric cancer but an ulcerating cancer may appear similar to a benign ulcer. If the tumour is widely infiltrating (linitis plastica) a typically immobile stomach is seen. Endoscopy may be the initial investigation or done only in those patients with abnormal barium meal results. During endoscopy, multiple biopsies and brushings for cytological examination are taken. This is especially important for the ulcerating cancer which may appear benign to the endoscopist.

Evidence for the presence of spread of any tumour is obtained both by clinical examination (e.g. lymph nodes in the neck) and by the use of chest X-ray, liver blood tests, upper abdominal ultrasound and/or CT scan.

Treatment

Surgery

Since the only hope of cure is surgical resection of the tumour, treatment is initially aimed at identifying those

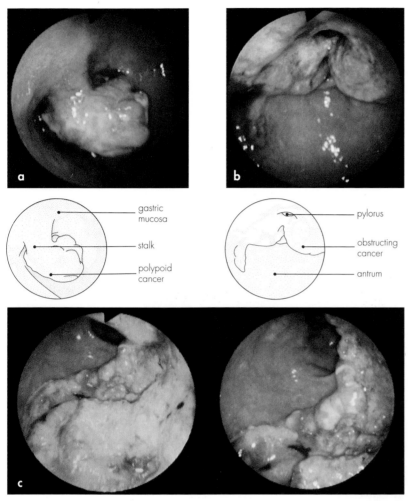

Fig. 3.13 a. Polypoid adenocarcinoma of the body of the stomach, which appears pedunculated, and **b** of the antrum, occluding the gastric outlet. **c.** Centrally ulcerated adenocarcinoma. The base of the ulcer is necrotic tumour, granulation tissue, and tumour nodules (left). Tumour nodules can be clearly seen at the distal rim of the ulcer (right). This would be an appropriate area for biopsy.

patients in whom this is feasible. A curative operation depends not only on resection of the diseased stomach by partial or total gastrectomy, but also on the removal of draining lymph nodes, including those immediately beyond the spread of disease.

When radical resection is not feasible, or is inappropriate due to the patient's general health, then palliation may be obtained by two methods:
• partial gastrectomy or gastroenterostomy may be appropriate, but total gastrectomy for proximal lesions is usually avoided;
• for tumours arising at the oesophagogastric junction, a prosthesis may be inserted endoscopically to maintain swallowing (Fig. 3.14).

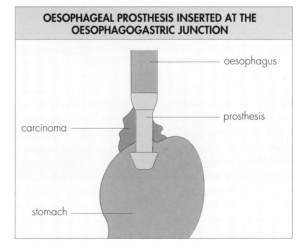

OESOPHAGEAL PROSTHESIS INSERTED AT THE OESOPHAGOGASTRIC JUNCTION

Fig. 3.14 An oesophageal prosthesis inserted at the oesophagogastric junction.

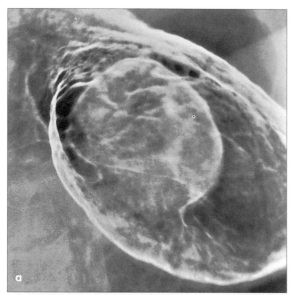

Fig. 3.15 Endoscopic laser coagulation. **a.** X-ray of gastric carcinoma in an elderly woman. **b.** Endoscopy revealed a large polypoid cancer in the cardia. The tumour was best seen on retroflexion. **c.** The tumour began to bleed while being inspected endoscopically. **d.** After partial laser therapy, the tumour had become smaller and there was no evidence of bleeding. **e.** Several weeks later, after more laser therapy, no cancer was seen. Only a small ulcer was noted in the area of treatment. **f.** Finally, the area was completely healed. Biopsy of the area was negative for residual tumour. The only abnormality was a slight retraction in the treatment area.

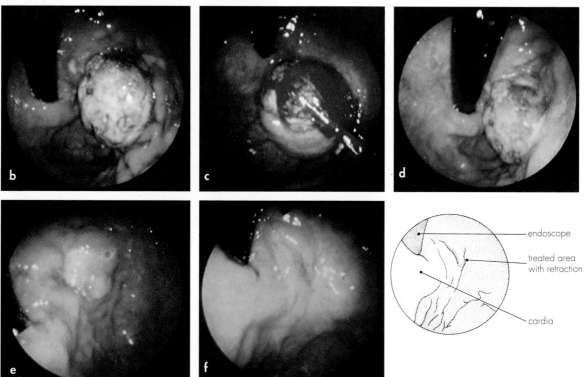

Endoscopic Therapy

Increasing use is being made of endoscopic laser therapy, or sclerotherapy, with absolute alcohol, to reduce obstructing tumour bulk or control bleeding (Fig. 3.15).

Other Approaches

Radiotherapy is not beneficial, but some regimes of combination chemotherapy can give useful remissions in approximately 30% of patients.

Prognosis

EGC has a favourable outcome with a 90% 5-year survival rate after surgery. The outcome in AGC is appalling and depends upon the depth of invasion and the extent of lymph node spread. Even in those undergoing a 'curative' resection, the 5-year survival rate is less than 25%, and for the majority of patients it is worse.

POINTS TO REMEMBER

- Consider endoscopy for any patient over 50 who presents with a first episode of epigastric pain
- Surgery for EGC is rare in western countries
- Surgery may be curative or provide good palliation
- Therapeutic endoscopy is increasingly being used to control bleeding

4. Small Intestinal Disease

INTRODUCTION

This chapter deals with the commoner conditions which affect the small intestine, but Crohn's disease and functional bowel disorders, which are covered in other chapters (6 and 7), are excluded.

The majority of small intestinal disorders share a modest number of symptoms. They can be broadly categorized into these which result from alterations in structure and obstruction of the intestinal lumen, and those which are due to malabsorption of various nutrients particularly fat. It is important to note that considerable malabsorption may occur in the absence of florid gastroenterological symptoms.

INTESTINAL OBSTRUCTION

The colicky pain is felt in the centre of the abdomen, is accompanied by borborygmi, and may be precipitated by food and relieved by vomiting. The vomitus becomes faeculent following bacterial overgrowth in distal obstruction. Distension is most marked in ileal obstruction. Figure 4.1 shows visible peristalsis in a thin patient, and multiple air/fluid levels are shown in Figure 4.2.

Obstruction is most frequently due to an extrinsic cause such as a strangulated hernia, adhesion or metastatic malignancy. The intestine may be occluded by an intraluminal mass such as polypoid tumour causing intussusception, or a large gall stone as in gall stone ileus. Strictures are common features in Crohn's disease, intestinal lymphoma and tuberculosis (Fig. 4.3).

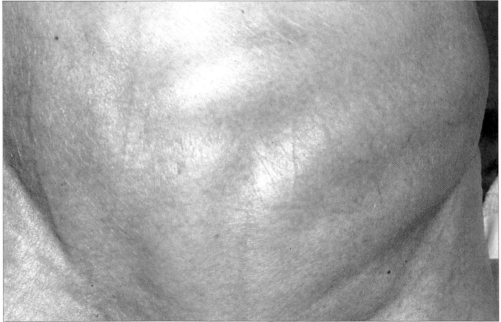

Fig. 4.1 A patient with bowel obstruction showing loops of distended small bowel. Peristalsis was visable.

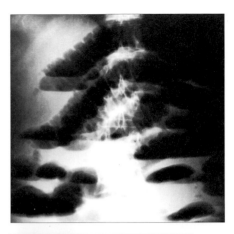

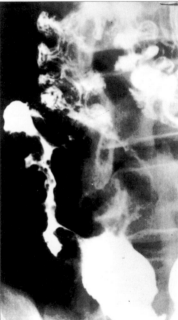

Fig. 4.2 Abdominal radiograph (erect view) showing multiple air/fluid levels in the small bowel due to obstruction.

valvulae
conniventes
in jejunum

multiple
air/fluid
levels

ileum

Fig. 4.3 Barium enema in hypertrophic tuberculosis, mainly affecting the ascending colon in a 32-year-old Indian presenting with a large mass in the right iliac fossa.

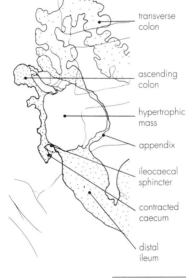

transverse
colon

ascending
colon

hypertrophic
mass

appendix

ileocaecal
sphincter

contracted
caecum

distal
ileum

MALABSORPTION

The typical features of the diarrhoea of malabsorption are due the poor digestion and absorption of fat and are given in Diagnosis below. A number of conditions can cause small intestinal malabsorption (Fig. 4.4). The appearance is non-specific and does not suggest any particular cause of the malabsorption. The stool is loose and greasy, adheres to the lavatory bowel, and is difficult to flush away. Unusually foul wind is a notable feature.

CAUSES OF SMALL INTESTINAL MALABSORPTION
coeliac disease/dermatitis herpetiformis
Crohn's disease
infective
tropical sprue
Whipple's disease
contaminated small bowel
lymphangiectasia
disaccharidase deficiency
intestinal resection

Fig. 4.4 Causes of small intestinal malabsorption.

NUTRITIONAL DEFICIENCIES IN MALABSORPTION		
Deficiency	**Results**	**Symptom**
calories	weight loss growth retardation	weight loss poor growth
protein	muscle wasting hypoproteinaemia and oedema	weakness ankle swelling
iron/folate	anaemia	tiredness and breathlessness
vitamin B_{12}	anaemia/subacute combined degeneration of the spinal cord	poor balance/sensation
vitamin D	osteomalacia (in adults) or rickets (in children)	bone pain (in adults) and deformity (in children)
vitamin K	reduced clotting factors	easy bruising and bleeding
vitamin C	blood vessel fragility	easy bruising and bleeding
vitamin A	poor night vision	may not be noticed
calcium and magnesium	neuromuscular upset	tetany and weakness
potassium	neuromuscular upset	weakness

Fig. 4.5 Nutritional deficiencies in malabsorption.

Although diarrhoea is a common presenting symptom, many patients have complaints which are due to one or more of the nutritional deficiencies that are a consequence of malabsorption. In young children, diarrhoea is often accompanied by failure to thrive, poor growth, abdominal distension and pain. The older child may experience delayed puberty in addition to weight loss and stunting of growth. Secondary amenorrhoea can be the presenting complaint in adolescent and adult females.

In adults, weight loss may be insidious or dramatic to the point of emaciation, depending on the underlying cause. Protein loss leads to hypoproteinaemia and oedema which may mask underlying muscle wasting. Iron and folic acid deficiency is common in jejunal disease but the terminal ileum must be affected before vitamin B_{12} malabsorption occurs in the presence of normal intrinsic factor production by the stomach. A lack of the fat-soluble vitamins A, D and K occurs. Hypovitaminosis A will cause poor night vision but is uncommon. More frequently, osteomalacia results from poor calcium utilization secondary to a lack of vitamin D. In children, the equivalent of osteomalacia is rickets, but this may not be apparent until the child is treated and the bones begin to grow again. A tendency to easy bruising and bleeding indicates a lack of vitamin K and/or vitamin C. Neuromuscular function may be disturbed by reduced potassium, calcium and magnesium levels. The nutritional consequences of malabsorption and their symptoms are summarized in Fig. 4.5. Figure 4.6 illustrates the typical radiological appearances in malabsorption.

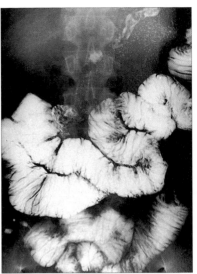

Fig. 4.6 Malabsorption pattern on barium follow-through. Malabsorption is indicated by widening of the jejual loops to a maximum of 5.4 cm (normal <3 cm). The valvulae conniventes across the loops are thickened.

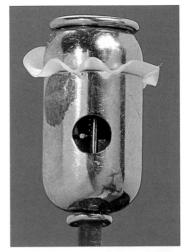

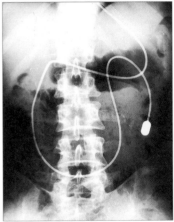

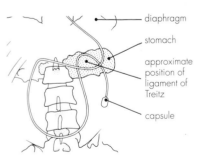

Fig. 4.7 A small intestinal biopsy capsule (upper) and a plain abdominal radiograph showing the capsule in the jejunum distal to the ligaments of Treitz (lower).

— diaphragm
— stomach
— approximate position of ligament of Treitz
— capsule

DIAGNOSIS

Symptoms of small intestine obstruction

- Colicky pain
- Borborygmi
- Vomiting
- Abdominal distension
- Visible peristalsis
- Fluid levels on X-rays

Malabsorption diarrhoea

- Pale
- Bulky
- Floats
- Offensive
- Flatulent

COELIAC DISEASE

Coeliac disease is the most common single cause of malabsorption in Europe and the USA. The prevalence of this condition varies greatly from 1/300 in parts of Ireland, through 1/1800 in the UK, to 1/6,500 in Scandinavia. It is much less common in the Far East.

PATHOGENESIS

Environmental

The mucosa of the small intestine is damaged by an immunological response to the water-insoluble protein, gluten. This is present in wheat, rye and barley. The term gluten enteropathy is a useful descriptive

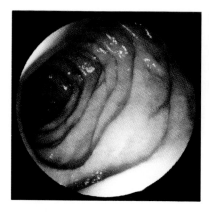

Fig. 4.8 Normal descending duodenum. Circular folds are seen.

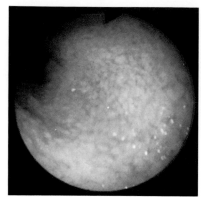

Fig. 4.9 Coeliac appearance of the duodenum. Close examination of the mucosa shows complete villous atrophy. Circular folds are absent.

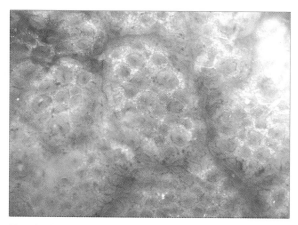

Fig. 4.10 Dissecting microscope appearance of a sub-total villous atrophy showing the mosaic pattern,

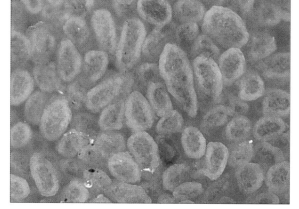

Fig. 4.11 Dissecting microscope appearance of jejunal mucosa showing normal finger-like villi.

synonym which accurately describes the condition. The toxicity of the gluten is related to a mixture of proteins, the α- and β-gliadins.

Genetic

There is a genetic component in coeliac disease. Ten per cent of first degree relatives have evidence of intestinal damage, even if they are asymptomatic. The risk of siblings or offspring developing coeliac disease is between 2 and 5%.

DIAGNOSIS

Gluten enteropathy may present with any combination of the symptoms of malabsorption described

above. The diagnosis can only confirmed by small intestinal biopsy. This can be obtained either by the use of a purpose-built small intestinal biopsy capsule as shown in Fig. 4.7 or via a standard gastroscope. In the latter cases it is important that the biopsy is taken from as far round the duodenum as possible, to avoid histological confusion with duodenitis. At endoscopy, the duodenal mucosa may appear atrophic with few circular folds. These appearances should raise the suspicion of coeliac disease in any patient who is being investigated for anaemia or malabsorption. Figures 4.8 and 4.9 show a normal duodenum and the coeliac appearance.

Biopsies are examined under an operating microscope and histologically. The villi are shortened in sub-total villous atrophy (Fig. 4.10) in comparison with their normal appearance (Fig. 4.11), and the mucosa appears flat. Normal histology and sub-total

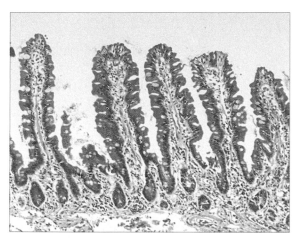

Fig. 4.12 Normal jejunal biopsy showing, tall finger-like villi.

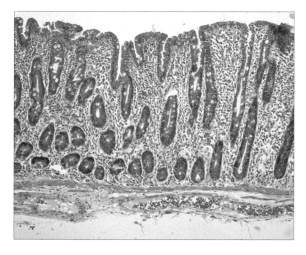

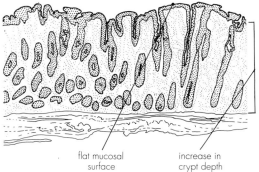

flat mucosal surface   increase in crypt depth

Fig. 4.13 Sub-total villous atrophy showing total absence of villi and a corresponding increase in depth of the crypts, producing an apparentley increased mucosal thickness. H & E, x70.

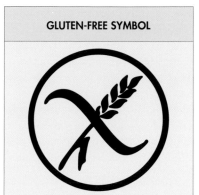

GLUTEN-FREE SYMBOL

Fig. 4.14 Symbol indicating that a food product is gluten-free.

villous atrophy are compared in Figs. 4.12 and 4.13. In the UK, a flat biopsy in an adult is virtually pathognomonic of coeliac disease. In children, allergy to cows' milk or soya protein may given similar appearances.

After adequate dietary treatment, usually for several months, a repeat biopsy must be obtained to demonstrate improvement. Children should have a third biopsy after gluten challenge because of the possible confusion with milk and soya allergies.

TREATMENT

The treatment is the removal of gluten from the diet. This means that all wheat, rye and barley products must be avoided for life. There is debate about whether oats should also be withdrawn. In western societies where bread is the staple carbohydrate source, a gluten-free diet involves a significant change in eating habits, or the re-education of the palate to gluten-free bread and biscuits. Many such products are now available on prescription in the UK, and many gluten-free foods are clearly marked, as in Fig. 4.14.

COMPLICATIONS

Benign ulceration and strictures of the small intestine occur rarely. It is impossible to distinguish clinically or radiologically between such lesions and the more sinister malignant complications, lymphoma and adenocarcinoma of the small intestine, and laparotomy is usually required. Lymphomas are usually derived from the T cell line, are often extensive (Fig 4.15) and respond poorly to chemotherapy and radiotherapy. Adenocarcinoma of the small bowel is found much more commonly in coeliac disease than in the normal population, but even in coeliacs it is unusual. Any deterioration in the stable condition of a patient known to have coeliac disease should prompt investigation for one of these complications. Strict adherence to a gluten-free diet probably reduces the likelihood of malignant change.

Other complications are commonly associated with inadequate treatment. This can lead to a recurrence of diarrhoea and persistent, low-grade malabsorption and deficiency states previously described.

DERMATITIS HERPETIFORMIS

Dermatitis herpetiformis is an intensely itchy, blistering skin condition (Fig. 4.16). The majority of patients with dermatitis herpetiformis have an enteropathy which responds to a gluten-free diet, and

by definition they have coeliac disease. The intestinal damage appears to be patchier in these individuals, and features of malabsorption are often mild or absent. It is not known why most people who have coeliac disease do not develop dermatitis herpetiformis.

INTESTINAL INFECTIONS

Infestation with the protozoan parasite *Giardia lamblia* is probably the most common infective cause of malabsorption in the UK. Infection is usually contracted from infected water supplies, and travellers are often affected, although a large number of patients are infected without foreign travel. The infection may be asymptomatic. In acute attacks there is abdominal pain, bloating and the passage of diarrhoea and excess flatus. Typical malabsorptive features may supervene.

Diagnosis is made by finding the parasite in jejunal aspirate or small intestinal biopsy specimens. The cysts are sometimes found in the stool, but their absence does not exclude infection. Treatment with

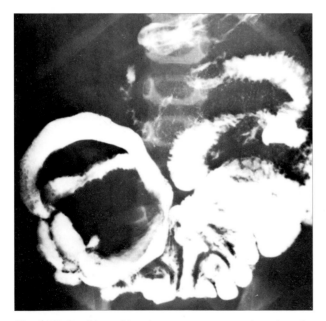

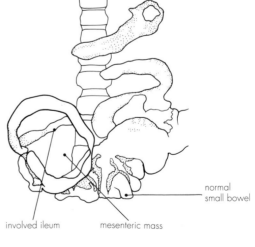

normal
small bowel

involved ileum   mesenteric mass

Fig. 4.15 Small bowel lymphoma in a patient with coeliac disease giving rise to a large mesenteric mass in the RIF. This is displacing and compressing several ileal loops which show effacement of the fold pattern and nodular irregularity, indicating musosal invasion.

metronidazole 2 g daily for three consecutive days, or a single dose of 2 g tinidazole is usually effective.

Other parasites such as *Stronglyoides stercoralis* may cause malabsorption. Infection is confined to tropical countries. Travellers may also contract hook-worm (*Ancylostoma duodenale* and *Nector ameri-canus*), roundworm (*Ascaris lumbracoides*) and tapeworm infections, from beef or pork, but none of these typically cause malabsorption. Infestation by the fish tapeworm *Diphyllobothrium latum* can cause B_{12} malabsorption.

TROPICAL SPRUE

This disease is restricted to the geographical regions shown in Fig. 4.17. This and its association with chronic diarrhoeal infections and bacterial overgrowth give rise to the synonymous title of post-infective tropical malabsorption. Travellers may return with a chronic malabsorptive diarrhoea, and it is essential that other commoner causes be excluded before a diagnosis of tropical sprue is made. The jejunal biopsy reveals partial villous atrophy which is patchier than in coeliac disease.

Treatment with tetracylcine 750 mg daily and folic acid 15 mg daily for four weeks is usually successful.

WHIPPLE'S DISEASE

This rare condition is due to an infective agent, possibly a streptococcus. The intestinal features may be preceded by years of mild arthritis. Some patients have depression, ophthalmoplegia, cardiac or neu-

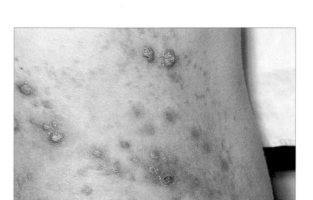

Fig. 4.16 Dermatitis hepetiformis. This skin disease presents with itchy plaques that blister. Almost all patients have small intestinal changes similar to coeliac disease and malabsoprtion can be demonstrated in some. Dapsone is used to control the cutaneous lesions. On a gluten-free diet the intestinal mucosa returns to normal and the dose of dapsone needed is much reduced or may no longer be required.

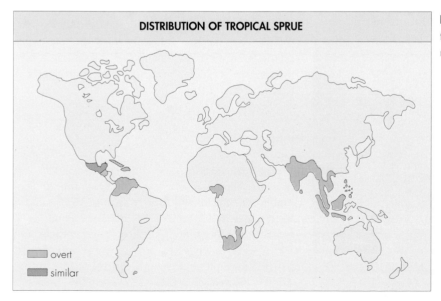

DISTRIBUTION OF TROPICAL SPRUE

overt

similar

Fig. 4.17 The distribution of tropical sprue and disorders resembling sprue.

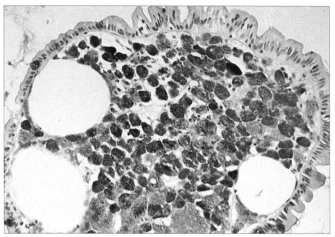
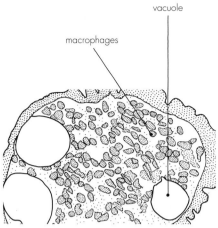

macrophages

vacuole

Fig. 4.18 The typical mucosal appearance in Whipple's disease. PAS-laden machrophages expanding the villus. Large vacuoles are also a characteristic finding. x180.

POSSIBLE CAUSES OF BACTERIAL CONTAMINATION	
Anatomical abnormality	**Functional failure**
jejunal diverticula	hypochlorhydria
postoperative complication	abnormal motility
fistulae	immune deficiency
intestinal obstruction	

Fig. 4.19 Possible causes of bacterial contamination.

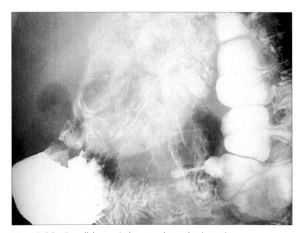

Fig. 4.20 Small bowel diverticula, which in this case are particularly large and numerous.

rological symptoms. Small bowel biopsy (Fig. 4.18) shows macrophages full of bacteria on periodic acid–Schiff (PAS) staining. Similar lesions may be found in the heart, lungs and brain.

Antibiotic treatment must be prolonged to effect a cure, and the neurological deficit may not completely resolve. Two weeks' treatment with penicillin and tetracycline is followed by tetracycline alone for six months or more, depending on response.

BACTERIAL CONTAMINATION

Also known as the blind loop or stagnant loop syndrome, bacterial contamination may be caused by one or more of a combination of anatomical abnormalities and a failure of one or more gastrointestinal functions (Fig. 4.19).

Causes

The normal small intestine contains relatively few organisms. They are fewest in the duodenum and jejunum where contaminants from ingested food are most frequent. In the distal ileum larger numbers of typical faecal flora, both anaerobes and aerobes, occur. A wide variety of bacteria have been implicated in the bacterial overgrowth syndrome, including *Escherichia coli*, *Klebsiella* and *Bacteroides* species.

Reservoirs of relatively stagnant intestinal fluid become colonized and intestinal function is compromised. Diverticula of the small intestine are commonest in the jejunum (Fig. 4.20). Single large diverticula are found in the duodenum, most frequently in the periampullary area, and rarely cause malabsorption. Ileal diverticula are less common. Potential blind loops may be created by surgery, vagotomy may reduce intestinal motility and gastric resection will lead to hypochlorhydria. Fistulae between the colon and small intestine or stomach will introduce faecal flora. Fistulae may occur as a postoperative complication or as a feature of Crohn's disease or gastrointestinal malignancy. The features of chronic obstruction may be mimicked by visceral myopathies or neuropathies which cause 'pseudo-obstruction' because of disordered motility, even though no physical obstruction exists.

Diagnosis

The history, abnormal blood tests and small bowel follow-though radiology will reveal the combination of circumstances likely to give rise to bacterial contamination. It is important to note that while the B_{12} level may be low as a result of bacterial use of the vitamin, folic acid levels may be high because some bacteria produce it.

Aspiration of secretions from the small intestine for culture is helpful. Many patients are elderly and frail, and the diagnosis can be confirmed by the use of a breath test using either ^{14}C-labelled glycocholate or glucose and hydrogen. In the former, the bacterial metabolism produces ^{14}C-labelled CO_2. This is exhaled and can be measured. In the latter, small doses of oral glucose are given. The bacteria produce excess hydrogen which can be detected in the expired air.

Treatment

Tetracycline and metronidazole are most useful, together with nutritional and vitamin supplements to correct specific deficiencies. The duration of treatment will vary depending on the response, and the rapidity of relapse after cessation of antibiotics. Initial recovery may require weeks or months of therapy. Lifelong treatment is sometimes necessary, using a rotating regime of different antibiotics to reduce the incidence of bacterial resistance.

LYMPHANGIECTASIA

Lymphangiectasia, dilatation of the lymph channels, may be either a rare primary condition which affects children and young adults, or a secondary phenomenon caused by obstruction to the thoracic duct or other major lymphatic channels. Any malignant infiltration may be implicated. Benign causes include constrictive pericarditis, retroperitoneal fibrosis, Crohn's disease and tuberculosis.

Patients may have few gastrointestinal symptoms. Leg oedema is a striking feature in adults, and pleural effusions and ascites are common due to a combination of hypoproteinaemia and lymphatic obstruction. Investigation will reveal increased protein loss from the intestine, and the small intestinal biopsy shows distorted villi with dilated lacteals (Fig. 4.21).

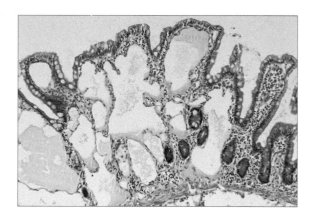

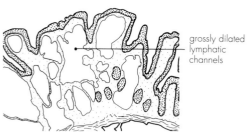

grossly dilated lymphatic channels

Fig. 4.21 Lymphangiectasia of the small bowel secondary to an obstructing carcinoma. H & E stain, x70.

Treatment

Dietary manipulation can be strikingly effective. Medium chain triglycerides, which are well absorbed without patent lymphatics, should be substituted for long chain fats. The reduced lymph flow resulting from this treatment leads to lower protein losses from the intestine. Fat-soluble vitamins and calcium supplements may be required.

DISACCHARIDASE DEFICIENCY

Deficiency of any mucosal disaccharidase will cause malabsorption of a specific sugar. The most important is alactasia. This is inherited as an autosomal recessive trait and affects between 5 and 15% of Northern European and North American whites. The prevalence in parts of Africa is 75–100%. Secondary lactase deficiency can follow mucosal damage in coeliac disease, Crohn's disease, tropical sprue and other intestinal infections. In these cases it is often reversible.

Symptoms are very variable, and milk may be suprisingly well tolerated. The diagnosis can be confirmed by a lactose tolerance test. After 50 g lactose, the blood glucose will fail to rise if lactase is absent. An alternative is to measure breath hydrogen after the lactose load. In this case there will be abnormal amounts of hydrogen excreted as the undigested lactose reaches the bacteria in the caecum. The enzyme activity can be measure in a small intestinal biopsy.

Treatment

Lactose-free diets will usually bring about a marked improvement in symptoms in primary hypolactasia. The amount of milk and milk products taken in the long term can then be adjusted to attain a suitable compromise between symptoms and dietary inconvenience. Secondary hypolactasia also responds to temporary lactose withdrawal while the precipitating cause is treated. It is important to remember that many phamaceutical tablets contain sufficient lactose to cause symptoms in those with lactase deficiency.

INTESTINAL RESECTION AND INTESTINAL FAILURE

The concept of intestinal failure is analogous to renal failure. There is a spectrum of insufficient intestinal function which becomes more significant as the length of intestine becomes shorter. Recurrent resections for Crohn's disease and massive resection for intestinal infarction due to either arterial or venous occlusion are the commonest causes of intestinal resection sufficient to result in intestinal failure. Scleroderma, visceral myopathy and neuropathy and extensive Crohn's disease may compromise intestinal function to the point where nutritional support as detailed below is required, even when significant intestinal resection has not been necessary.

Effects and Management of Resection

The small intestine measures between 2 and 3 m in life. The proximal 40% is jejunum, the remainder ileum. Over 90% of ingested protein, carbohydrate and fat has been absorbed by the time the chyme has traversed the first metre of jejunum. The remainder of the small intestine is responsible for the reabsorption of secreted digestive juices, minerals and water. There is thus a great reserve of absorptive capacity and most resections cause no change in intestinal function. However, the jejunum and proximal item cannot adapt to take over the specialized functions of the terminal ileum to absorb vitamin B_{12} and bile salts; Fig. 4.22 illustrates the consequences of terminal ileal resection.

The effects of substantial small bowel resection depend to an extent on whether the colon has been retained. If it has, then the salt and water balance is easier to maintain than if there is an ileostomy or a jejunostomy, in which cases there is an unavoidable daily loss of water and electrolytes which has to be replaced. However, the colon may be irritated by excess bile acids and fatty acids which cause troublesome diarrhoea. When less than 150 cm of small intestine remains, malabsorption of all nutrients is likely. A constant proportion of all foods will be absorbed regardless of whether the proteins, carbohydrates and fats are given in solid, liquid or predigested elemental diets. It is important to recognize that increased total amounts of nutrients are necessary, together with appropriate vitamin supplements. Some patients will benefit from a low-fat diet, but this is by no means necessary for all, and indeed the reduced calorie intake can be detrimental. Large amounts of fluid should be avoided at mealtimes in an effort to slow intestinal transit times. Antidiarrhoeal agents such as codeine phosphate, loperamide and diphenoxylate are also worth a trial, although response is variable.

Patients with a short length of residual intestine will need regular monitoring by a specialized hospital unit. The least severely affected need no food supplement but may require treatment with oral rehydration solutions to replace water and electrolyte losses. When necessary, supplementary liquid food preparations can be given either as oral sip feeds or by nasogastric tube overnight, to boost the total daily food intake. In the extreme case, where so little intestine remains that adequate nourishment is impossible despite these measures, parenteral feeding offers survival and an acceptable quality of life for those who are otherwise healthy. All of these techniques can be learned by the patient, and allow independent life in their own home. Several hundred patients have received home parenteral nutrition in

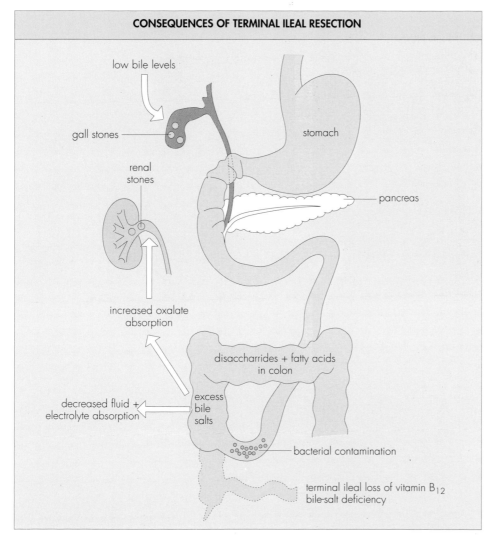

CONSEQUENCES OF TERMINAL ILEAL RESECTION

low bile levels

gall stones

renal stones

stomach

pancreas

increased oxalate absorption

disaccharides + fatty acids in colon

decreased fluid + electrolyte absorption

excess bile salts

bacterial contamination

terminal ileal loss of vitamin B_{12} bile-salt deficiency

Fig. 4.22
Consequences of terminal ileal esection.

the UK, the USA, Canada and European countries. Small intestinal transplantation is not yet a therapeutic option.

POINTS TO REMEMBER

Malabsorption

- Malabsorption can occur without diarrhoea
- Malabsorption must be considered in any child with poor growth or development

Coeliac disease

- Coeliac disease is the commonest cause of malabsorption in the West
- A small bowel biopsy is essential to confirm coeliac disease
- The commonest complication of coeliac disease is inadvertant non-compliance with the gluten-free diet
- Deterioration in a previoulsy stable coeliac may indicate malignancy

5. Disorders of the Pancreas and Extrahepatic Biliary Tree

PANCREATIC CARCINOMA

Epidemiology

Adenocarcinoma of the pancreas is increasing in frequency. It occurs predominantly in those over the age of 65 and is commoner in men. The annual incidence of pancreatic cancer in the USA is between 150 and 200 per million, and it accounts for nearly 5% of all cancer deaths. Carcinoma of the pancreas is associated with cigarette smoking and previous partial gastrectomy. Despite much interest, there is no convincing data showing that coffee consumption or alcohol are implicated.

Pathogenesis

Two thirds of pancreatic tumours arise in the head of the pancreas. Carcinomas arising in this region may

be difficult to distinguish from those arising within the lower common bile duct or the ampulla of Vater (Fig. 5.1). Jaundice is usually an early feature.

Tumours arising in the body or tail of the pancreas have generally invaded local structures by the time of presentation. In this case, jaundice is a much later feature. The typical sites of spread of the tumour are shown in Fig. 5.2.

Prognosis

The outlook remains bleak. A curative procedure (Whipple's operation – pancreatico-duodenectomy) is appropriate for small tumours in young patients (see Fig. 5.3). Even in this small group, the mean survival is less than two years with considerable perioperative mortality.

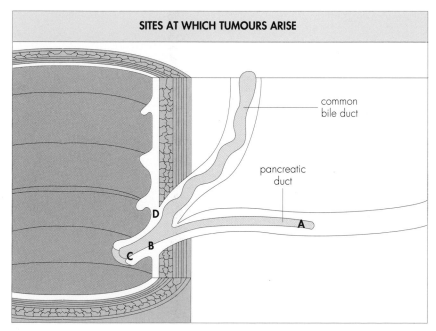

SITES AT WHICH TUMOURS ARISE

common bile duct

pancreatic duct

Fig. 5.1 Representation of the ampulla of Vater and associated strictures. Tumours in this region arise most commonly from the pancreatic duct or its branches in the head of the pancreas (A), but also can arise in the ampulla itself (B), in the duodenal mucosa, particularly at its junction with the ampulla (C), or in the common bile duct (D).

ADENOCARCINOMA OF THE PANCREAS

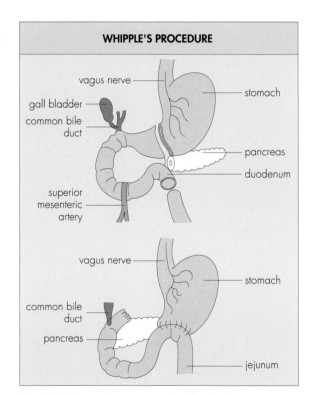

	Spread	Symptoms
	duodenum	pain, vomiting, obstruction
	bile duct and pancreas	jaundice, pancreatitis
	retroperitoneum	back pain
	spleen and colon	left upper quadrant pain
	portal and splenic veins	varices, splenomegaly, hepatic disorders
	peritoneal cavity	ascites
	lymph nodes	obstructive jaundice
	blood stream	distant metastases

Fig. 5.2 Sites of spread and production of symptoms in adenocarcinoma of the pancreas.

WHIPPLE'S PROCEDURE

Fig. 5.3 Schematic representation of radical pancreatico-duodenectomy (Whipple's procedure). The organs removed include the distal stomach, the whole of the duodenum, the first part of the jejunum and the end part of the body of the pancreas.

DIAGNOSIS

Symptoms and features

Systemic features
• Weight loss
• Weakness
• Thrombophlebitis migrans

Biliary obstruction
• Jaundice
• Hepatomegaly
• Palpable gall bladder

Local invasion
• Pain
• Duodenal obstruction
• Anaemia
• Obstruction of pancreatic duct with steatorrhoea and glycosuria
• Splenic and portal vein thrombosis with splenomegaly

Metastatic disease
• Distant sites, e.g. liver, lung
• Left supraclavicular lymph node

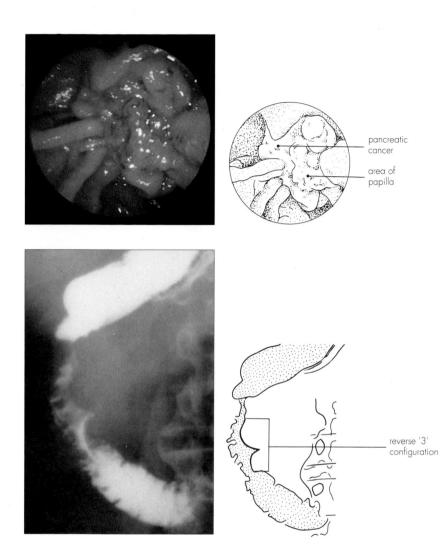

Fig. 5.4 A pancreatic carcinoma has invaded the duodenal wall just above the papilla. The folds are irregular and nodular.

pancreatic cancer

area of papilla

Fig. 5.5 The medial border of the duodenal C-loop has a classic reverse '3' configuration, correlating with a tumour originating in the head of the pancreas, with secondary involvement of ampullary structures.

reverse '3' configuration

The typical symptoms of pancreatic carcinoma are shown opposite. Which of them predominates will depend largely on the exact anatomical location of the tumour. Thus, a tumour arising in the head of the pancreas is likely to present with jaundice whilst a tumour arising in the body or tail will present with pain and weight loss. The pain of pancreatic carcinoma may be severe and often radiates to the back. Pancreatic pain may sometimes be relieved by sitting forward. Both diabetes mellitus and steatorrhoea may occur, but malabsorption is uncommon.

Investigation

In the absence of jaundice, diagnosing pancreatic carcinoma relies on a high index of suspicion, as many of the other symptoms are not specific. Blood tests are not diagnostic and chest X-rays seldom reveal any abnormality. Duodenal compression may be seen at endoscopy and, occasionally, direct extension of the tumour into the duodenal wall will allow diagnosis (Fig. 5.4). A barium meal may show widening of the duodenal loop, indicating an obstructive pancreatic mass (Fig. 5.5).

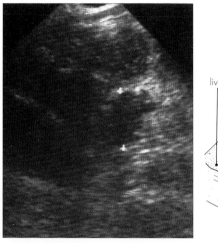
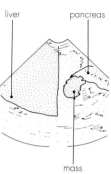

Fig.5.6 Pancreatic mass causing obstructive jaundice.

liver
pancreas
mass

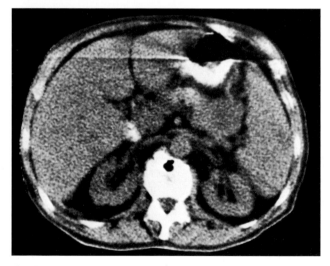
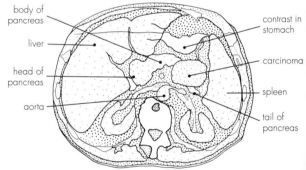

body of pancreas
liver
head of pancreas
aorta
contrast in stomach
carcinoma
spleen
tail of pancreas

Fig. 5.7 CT scan appearance of a pancreatic carcinoma.

Ultrasound is the appropriate initial investigation, particularly if jaundice is present (Fig. 5.6). Unfortunately, bowel gas may sometimes obscure the pancreas and then a CT scan is performed (Fig. 5.7). With either technique, a pancreatic mass may be identified. A biopsy or fine needle aspiration may be diagnostic in up to 75% of patients with pancreatic carcinoma. Endoscopic retrograde cholangiopancreatography (ERCP) is complementary and enables visualization of both the pancreatic (Fig. 5.8) and biliary tracts (Fig. 5.9). ERCP has the additional advantage that palliative relief of jaundice may be provided by the same technique (see below).

Treatment

For most patients palliative treatment is all that can be offered. In the younger, fitter patients, surgical palliation by choledochojejunostomy and gastroenterostomy is appropriate. In elderly, frail patients, endoscopic or percutaneous transhepatic biliary endoprosthesis (stent) insertion is used to relieve jaundice. Stents are inserted over a guidewire and catheter, which are passed through the stricture or occlusion of the bile duct (Fig. 5.10), which provide rapid relief from jaundice (Fig. 5.11). They are likely to become blocked after a few months, by debris or

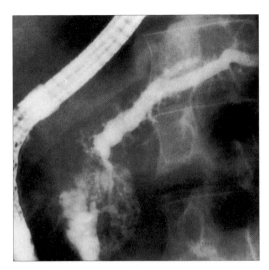

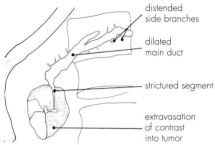

Fig. 5.8 ERCP showing a stricture of the pancreatic duct due to carcinoma of the head of the pancreas.

distended side branches

dilated main duct

strictured segment

extravasation of contrast into tumor

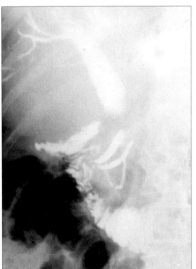

Fig. 5.9 Pancreatic carcinoma. A carcinoma has completely obstructed the pancreatic duct and partially blocked the bile duct. Although the biliary stricture cannot be clearly seen, the dilated proximal duct has filled.

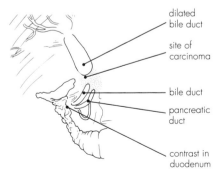

dilated bile duct

site of carcinoma

bile duct

pancreatic duct

contrast in duodenum

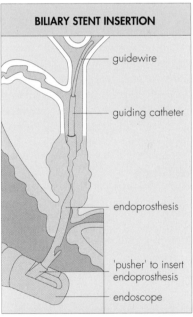

BILIARY STENT INSERTION

guidewire

guiding catheter

endoprosthesis

'pusher' to insert endoprosthesis

endoscope

Fig. 5.10 Method of endoscopic biliary endoprosthesis (stent) insertion.

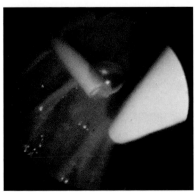

Fig. 5.11 Here, the stent is shown being separated from the pusher tube with bile emerging from the tip of the stent.

CONDITIONS ASSOCIATED WITH ACUTE PANCREATITIS

gall stones
alcohol abuse ⎤ account for up to 90% of cases
unknown ⎦

hyperlipidaemia
hypercalcaemia
trauma
renal failure
intraductal parasites
drugs, e.g. azathioprine
following ERCP
? pancreas divisum

Fig. 5.12 Conditions associated with acute pancreatitis.

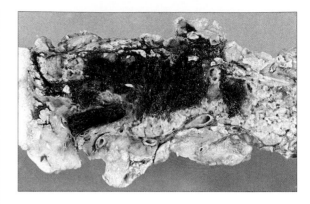

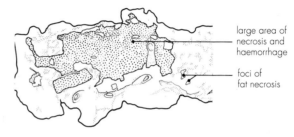

large area of
necrosis and
haemorrhage

foci of
fat necrosis

Fig. 5.13 The macroscopic appearance in acute haemorrhagic pancreatitis showing a large area of parenchymal necrosis and haemorrhage.

tumour, and then require replacement. The mean survival, once jaundice has occurred in pancreatic cancer, is six months or less, but relief of jaundice and pruritis can markedly improve the quality of life. The other manifestations of unresectable pancreatic carcinoma are treated symptomatically, but remorseless deterioration is inevitable.

POINTS TO REMEMBER

• Curative surgery should be considered in younger, fitter patients presenting with jaundice
• Effective palliation of jaundice is possible for the majority of patients
• Mean survival is less than 1 year

PANCREATITIS

Introduction

Pancreatitis may be acute or chronic. Although attacks of acute pancreatitis are of variable severity, there is usually complete recovery of endocrine and exocrine functions between attacks. Chronic pancreatitis, however, is an insidious, progressive disease, frequently with exacerbations identical to attacks of acute pancreatitis. Distinguishing between an exacerbation of chronic pancreatitis and an attack of acute pancreatitis may not be possible during the acute illness. The treatment for an acute attack is the same, and the true diagnosis becomes clear from the subsequent course of the disease.

Previous terms such as relapsing acute pancreatitis and chronic relapsing pancreatitis are no longer used.

ACUTE PANCREATITIS

Epidemiology
Data from the USA and England suggest that there is an annual incidence of approximately 10/100,000. The disease occurs equally in men and women and the incidence rises with age. A higher incidence has been reported from Denmark but the data was collected in a different way and may not be comparable to the previous studies.

The initial attack of acute pancreatitis has a greater mortality rate than recurrent attacks.

Pathogenesis

Acute pancreatitis occurs when proteolytic enzymes are activated within the pancreas, leading to auto-digestion. There are a variety of causes for this activation, the most common ones being alcohol and gall stones (Fig. 5.12). Obstruction of the pancreatic duct by carcinoma, reflux of duodenal contents and bile have all been cited as other causes, or there may be no recognizable cause at all. However, the pathological mechanisms which lead to acute pancreatitis are not clearly understood.

DIAGNOSIS

Symptoms and features

Acute pancreatitis
Early
- Epigastric or left-sided hypochondrial pain, which is usually continuous and radiates to the back
- Nausea and vomiting
- Fever
- Hypotension

Late
- Adult respiratory distress syndrome (ARDS)
- Acute tubular necrosis
- Disseminated intravascular coagulation (DIC)
- Hyperglycaemia
- Discoloration of the flanks (Grey Turner's sign; rare)
- Periumbilical discolouration (Cullen's sign; rare)
- Subcutaneous fat necrosis

An 'acute abdomen' is presented with more specific signs developing later. It is vital to recognize that the severity of attacks of acute pancreatitis may range from the mild (where the pancreas is oedematous, the inflammatory process is confined to the gland, and recovery is rapid) to the severe attack with widespread necrosis (Fig. 5.13) and life-threatening multisystem involvement.

Investigations

Other acute abdominal conditions such as a perforated

FEATURES OF SEVERE ACUTE PANCREATITIS
white blood cell count >16,000 cells/mm^3
haematocrit falls by >10%
rising blood urea
acidosis
hypoxia
rising blood sugar
falling serum calcium
falling serum albumin

Fig. 5.14 Features of severe acute pancreatitis. Three or more positive findings correlate with a severe attack.

viscus or mesenteric ischaemia need to be excluded The serum amylase is characteristically elevated. Almost any abdominal emergency will produce a modest rise in the serum amylase and, in order to be diagnostic, the level must be elevated to more than five times the upper limit of the normal laboratory range. Hyperlipidaemia or macroamylasaemia may mislead diagnosis on rare occasions. If there is associated hyperlipidemia then serum amylase activity may be found to be normal whereas urinary amylase activity may be elevated. In the rare cases of macroamylasaemia, the patient is usually well despite a very high amylase level but there is little urinary amylase activity.

A plain abdominal X-ray and an erect chest X-ray are of value to help exclude other possible diagnoses, and may also show a localized ileus with dilated loops of small bowel (a 'sentinel' loop).

It is possible to accurately predict the severity of an attack of acute pancreatitis within the first 48 hours, should three or more of the features shown in Fig. 5.14 prove positive.

Treatment

Many attempts at specific therapy to modify the course of the disease have been made but none of them has been of any benefit in clinical trials. Treatment is largely supportive. In a mild attack, the patient will need analgesia and intravenous fluids; the attack subsides after a few days and oral intake can be recommenced. The treatment of severe attacks of acute pancreatitis is dependent upon the close monitoring of the patient's general condition together with urea and electrolytes, serum calcium, arterial blood gases, blood sugar and blood count. Total parenteral nutrition may be required and facilities for ventilatory support should be available. Such patients are best managed in a high dependency unit or intensive care unit.

Unless the aetiology of the pancreatitis is known, attempts should be made to identify gall stones at an early stage because this may influence subsequent treatment. An ultrasound examination of the gall bladder, liver, extrahepatic bile ducts and pancreas should be performed. Gall stone pancreatitis is treated by cholecystectomy once the attack has settled. Urgent ERCP and sphincterotomy is indicated for a severe attack of gall stone pancreatitis that does not settle. A pancreatic abscess may be life threatening and can complicate any severe attack of acute pancreatitis. These abscesses must be drained.

In rare cases with massive necrotizing pancreatitis, which is best seen on a CT scan, urgent subtotal pancreatectomy may be indicated despite the high mortality rate of the procedure in a severely ill individual.

The widespread use of ultrasound has revealed that pseudocyst formation is common. Small cysts may resolve spontaneously but larger cysts usually require drainage, either surgically into the stomach or adjacent bowel, or by ultrasound guided percutaneous drainage.

Prognosis

Good supportive care is essential but the overall mortality remains at approximately 10%. Several complications may arise (Fig. 5.15) but the increased use of abdominal ultrasound and CT scanning allows them to be identified at an early stage. These complications are associated with increased mortality.

CHRONIC PANCREATITIS

Epidemiology

There is little reliable data but figures from the USA and Denmark suggest an annual incidence of between 3.5 and 4/100,000, with the median age of onset being in the late 40s. The importance of alcohol cannot be overemphasized; an increasing incidence of

chronic pancreatitis can be expected as the average annual consumption of alchohol continues to rise.

Pathogenesis

There have been several attempts to define different types of chronic pancreatitis. There is a progressive sclerosing process which is usually insidious. In alcoholic chronic pancreatitis, which accounts for as much as 90% of cases in some western countries, it is thought that protein plugs are deposited in the small pancreatic ducts. These may calcify and lead to ectasia, atrophy and fibrosis. Attacks of acute pancreatitis may occur during the course of the disease but this is by no means inevitable. There is little evidence that the other causes of acute pancreatitis (see Fig. 5.12) lead to chronic pancreatitis. There may be focal damage after pancreatic trauma, and there is some evidence that pancreas divisum, a congenital anomaly, may be associated with chronic pancreatitis in the dorsal pancreas, which drains through the accessory papilla. In a significant minority of patients, the cause of chronic pancreatitis remains unknown.

DIAGNOSIS

Symptoms

Chronic pancreatitis
- Pain
- Diabetes mellitus
- Malabsorption and weight loss
- Obstructive jaundice
- Pancreatic pseudocyst

Chronic pancreatitis usually presents with any of the symptoms shown above. The diagnosis may be obvious in the alcoholic, with recurrent attacks of acute pancreatitis, but is more difficult to ascertain in many

COMPLICATIONS OF ACUTE PANCREATITIS

pseudocyst formation
pancreatic abscess formation
gastrointestinal bleeding
jaundice due to compression of the common bile duct

Fig. 5.15 Complications of acute pancreatitis.

patients. Also, distinguishing chronic pancreatitis from pancreatic carcinoma may be particularly difficult even after the appropriate investigations have been carried out.

Investigations

In the absence of jaundice or malabsorption, routine laboratory blood tests are normal. A plain abdominal X-ray may demonstrate pancreatic calcification which, when seen, is virtually diagnostic (Fig. 5.16).

There has been considerable interest in the development of tests of pancreatic exocrine function but, as yet, these tests lack both sensitivity and specificity and are therefore not routinely used. Evidence of malabsorption may be sought as outlined in Chapter 4.

Ultrasound examination of the pancreas may reveal an enlarged pancreatic duct, or distortion of the gland, but may otherwise be normal. An abdominal CT scan should be requested if the pancreas cannot be seen clearly by ultrasound. Both CT scanning and ultrasound are invaluable for the diagnosis of pancreatic pseudocysts (Fig. 5.17). ERCP is frequently

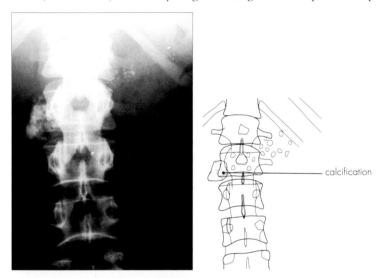

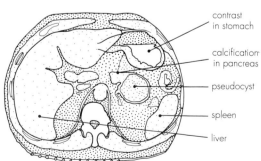

Fig. 5.16 Plain abdominal radiograph demonstrating extensive calcification in the duct system of a patient with chronic calcific pancreatitis due to alcoholism.

calcification

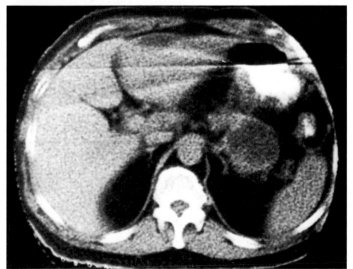

contrast in stomach

calcification in pancreas

pseudocyst

spleen

liver

Fig. 5.17 CT scan in chronic calcific pancreatitis showing a pseudocyst in the tail of the pancreas.

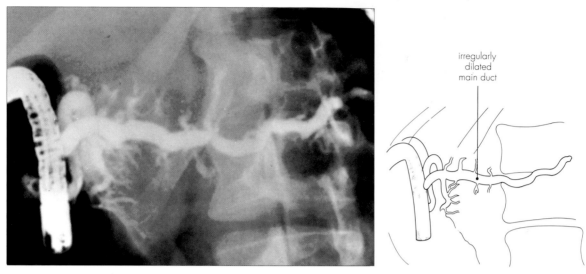

irregularly
dilated
main duct

Fig. 5.18 ERCP showing severe chronic pancreatitis (gross irregularity of side branches and irregular dilatation of pancreatic duct).

diagnostic, with a pancreatogram showing the typical dilatation and beading of the pancreatic duct (Fig. 5.18).

Treatment and Management

Patients should be persuaded to avoid alcohol even though they may find it an effective method of pain control! Malabsorption is treated with a low fat diet and oral pancreatic enzyme supplements. The latter may be combined with an H_2-receptor antagonist to prevent enzyme inactivation by gastric acid. Alternatively, pancreatic enzyme supplements may be given that are coated with a polymer which dissolves when the pH in the small bowel exceeds 6. Some patients also benefit from the use of oral medium chain triglycerides (MCT), which are partly water soluble and are readily absorbed without the need for pancreatic lipase. If diabetes mellitus occurs then conventional treatment is used; but insulin should be avoided if possible, since hypoglycaemia is frequent.

The major difficulty in the management of chronic pancreatitis is related to pain control. Non-steroidal anti-inflammatory drugs and simple analgesics should be tried initially, together with abstinence from alcohol. Many patients require opiates, but it should be remembered that in using these there is a considerable risk of dependence. Acupuncture and transcutaneous electric nerve stimulation (TENS) do not consistently provide benefit. A coeliac plexus nerve block may be attempted using alcohol to destroy the nerves; however, serious complications can occur, thus the procedure is not widely used. Short-term relief is sometimes produced by injecting corticosteroids with a local anaesthetic instead of alcohol. Fortunately, the pain of chronic pancreatitis tends to become less severe with time but this may take years. For some individuals surgical resection of part of the gland or, more commonly, a drainage procedure, such as a longitudinal pancreaticojejunostomy, should be considered.

Pancreatic pseudocysts occur commonly and, in many instances, can be left alone. If they become infected or exert pressure upon the stomach or biliary tree, then surgical drainage should be performed; usually internally into the stomach or jejunum. Occasionally, haemorrhage into a pseudocyst may occur and this is usually treated surgically or by embolization.

CHOLANGIOCARCINOMA

Carcinoma of the bile ducts may occur at any site. It is rare but is being increasingly recognized with the advent of better imaging techniques. It is more common in patients with congenital biliary disease, such as a choledochal cyst or polycystic disease of the liver, and it is associated with chronic liver fluke infestation in the Far East. It presents with progressive obstructive jaundice and, as a result, pancreatic carcinoma is generally and mistakenly suspected. Differentiation from a benign bile duct stricture may be occasionally difficult, although cytology obtained at the time of ERCP may be diagnostic. Surgical resection is dependent on the exact location of the tumour. After careful assessment, resection is usually feasible in only 20% of cases. In the majority of patients, palliation by the insertion of biliary stents is all that can be offered. Unfortunately, chemotherapy and irradiation (internal or external) have not increased the mean rate of survival which is less than six months.

SCLEROSING CHOLANGITIS

This is an uncommon disease of the bile ducts which may affect any part of the biliary tree. It usually involves both the extrahepatic and intrahepatic bile ducts and leads to areas of narrowing. The aetiology of the condition is unknown but assumed to be auto-immune. Affected individuals are more likely to be human leucocyte antigen (HLA) B8 or DR3 positive. There is a strong association with ulcerative colitis but the course of the disease is not affected by the colitis. Patients present with pruritus and jaundice. The asymptomatic stage of the disease is being increasingly identified in patients with ulcerative colitis who are found to have an isolated elevation of their alkaline phosphatase. The diagnosis is established by ERCP which shows characteristic beading of the bile ducts and 'pruning' of the intrahepatic ducts. The course of the disease is highly variable and drug treatment appears ineffective. Tight strictures of the extrahepatic bile ducts may be dilated and biliary stents sometimes inserted to maintain drainage. Occasionally, hepatic transplantation is required.

Some patients with the acquired immunodeficiency syndrome (AIDS) develop jaundice and are found to have cholangiographic appearances similar to those seen in sclerosing cholangitis. These patients usually have cryptosporidiosis or cytomegalovirus infection. It is assumed that the bile duct abnormalities result from bile duct infection but the mechanism is unknown. Treatment is symptomatic, and endoscopic sphincterotomy or biliary stent insertion are only rarely needed.

6. Inflammatory Bowel Disease

INTRODUCTION

Inflammatory bowel disease includes ulcerative colitis and Crohn's disease. These two conditions have important similarities and differences in their presenting features, clinical course, and medical and surgical treatment. In Europe and the USA, ulcerative colitis is more common, with a prevalence of between 80 and 100/100,000 per annum and an incidence of new cases of approximately 10/100,000 per annum. The figures for Crohn's disease are approximately half these, although the incidence of new cases is increasing.

Pathogenesis

Genetics

There is a greater incidence of inflammatory bowel disease within the families of existing sufferers than would normally be expected if left to chance. The theory of inheritance is complex and details have not been clarified. The risk is greater for the offspring of those with Crohn's disease compared to those with ulcerative colitis. It is not unusual for both diseases to occur in the same family.

Infection

It has been suspected that both ulcerative colitis and Crohn's disease are due to infective agents, but no consistent evidence exists to prove this. Current interest centres around the role of cell-wall deficient bacteria and atypical mycobacteria.

Psychosocial

Although ulcerative colitis was at one time thought to be a psychosomatic illness, no consistent evidence has been found to confirm this hypothesis. However, it is not uncommon for patients to relate relapses of their colitis symptoms to times of stress or major life events. Many patients have both inflammatory bowel disease and an irritable bowel syndrome. The important clinical distinction must be made between a true relapse of inflammatory bowel disease, and coexistent functional bowel symptoms.

Diet

There is no definite link between diet and the onset of inflammatory bowel disease. A number of patients develop a temporary inability to digest lactose after an acute attack: they may thus benefit from the avoidance of milk and milk products. There is no

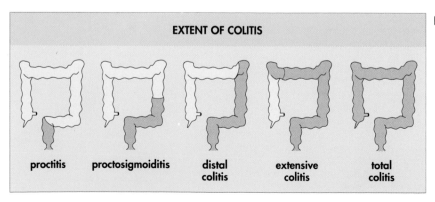

EXTENT OF COLITIS

proctitis | proctosigmoiditis | distal colitis | extensive colitis | total colitis

Fig. 6.1 Extent of colitis.

evidence that a true allergy to milk protein is a causative factor in ulcerative colitis.

Vascular

The small blood vessels, in areas affected by Crohn's disease, become damaged and occluded. This leads to ischaemia which may be part of the mechanism of ulceration. The stimulus for blood vessel damage has yet to be identified.

DIAGNOSIS

Symptoms

Ulcerative colitis: affects the colon
Proctitis
- Fresh blood and mucus passed alone
- Explosive wind
- Urgency

Proctosigmoiditis and distal colitis
- Blood mixed with faeces
- Malaise/lethargy
- Discomfort in the left iliac fossa or suprapubic area

Extensive and total colitis
- Liquid stools mixed with blood
- Stools often passed more than 10 times daily
- Weight loss
- Anaemia
- Fever
- Abdominal pain

Crohn's disease: can affect any part of the GI tract
- Swelling of lips
- Mouth ulcers
- Pain in the right iliac fossa
- Bowel looseness
- Anorexia
- Weight loss
- Anaemia
- Malabsorption
- Steatorrhoea (rare)
- Anal skin tags
- Anal fissuring and ulceration

Ulcerative Colitis

The severity of symptoms depends to a great extent on the proportion of the colon involved. It is convenient to consider attacks as being mild, moderate or severe, but this should be combined with an attempt to decide how much of the colon is involved, as this will influence the treatment (Fig. 6.1). Ulcerative colitis almost always involves the rectum and spreads proximally, in continuity. When normal mucosa is reached in ulcerative colitis, the remainder of the colon can confidently be expected to be normal.

Proctitis

Proctitis is the term used when the disease is limited to the rectum. The upper limit can be reached with the rigid sigmoidoscope and normal mucosa is visible proximally (Fig. 6.2). Rectal bleeding consists of fresh blood often passed alone or with mucus, often in the absence of stool. There is often great urgency in the need to defaecate, and evacuation is frequently

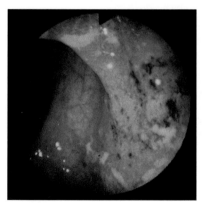

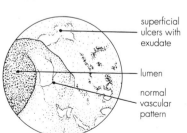

superficial ulcers with exudate

lumen

normal vascular pattern

Fig. 6.2 Sharp transition from normal to inflamed bowel is discernible at the rectosigmoid junction. Erythema and superficial ulceration of diseased mucosa contrasts with the normal vascular pattern.

explosive with copious wind. The patient may complain of 'diarrhoea' because of the need to visit the lavatory frequently, but a careful history will reveal that the stool is formed and passed relatively infrequently. There is little constitutional upset, but great

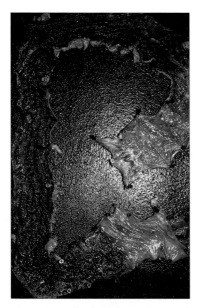

Fig. 6.3 Total colectomy specimen of severe ulcerative colitis.

ANATOMICAL FEATURES OF CROHN'S DISEASE

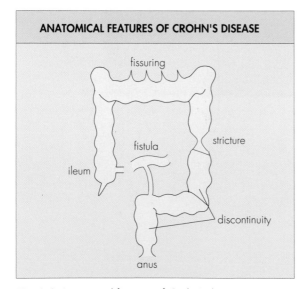

Fig. 6.4 Anatomical features of Crohn's disease.

social inconvenience and embarrassment are often the patient's greatest concern.

Proctosigmoiditis and Distal Colitis

The term proctosigmoiditis is sometimes used for disease limited to the rectum and sigmoid colon. Distal colitis or left-sided colitis are terms used to describe disease which extends from the rectum to the splenic flexure. The symptoms of proctitis coexist with the addition of a looser stool passed more frequently. Blood loss is often darker and mixed with the faeces. Constitutional symptoms, malaise and lethargy, are more common. Abdominal discomfort in the left iliac fossa or suprapubic area is often troublesome and is promptly relieved by bowel evacuation.

Extensive and Total Colitis

When colitis extends to the transverse colon, the terms substantial or extensive colitis are used. Total colitis indicates involvement from rectum to caecum (Fig. 6.3). Severe attacks are characterized by profuse liquid stools intimately mixed with blood, passed more than 15 times daily and often at night. There is weight loss, anaemia, fever and abdominal pain, although pain may be relatively unimpressive compared with the severity of the disease. Such an attack is potentially life-threatening. Urgent in-patient treatment, under the care of an appropriate specialist, is essential.

Crohn's Disease

Crohn's disease can affect any part of the gastrointestinal tract from the mouth to the anus, and in this it differs greatly from ulcerative colitis. The symptoms relate to the area involved and are thus much more varied, making the diagnosis more difficult to confirm (Fig. 6.4).

Oral Symptoms

Oral involvement may initially present as a swelling of the lips (Fig. 6.5) or irregularity of the gums. Mouth ulcers may be typically aphthoid (Fig. 6.6). In other cases, chronic, deep, irregular ulcers cause considerable discomfort and are difficult to eradicate. The oral lesions may antedate any intestinal involvement.

Oesophageal and Gastric Symptoms

Oesophageal and gastric Crohn's disease is uncommon. Duodenal involvement may initially be mistaken for resistant peptic ulcer disease until histology is obtained. Duodenal stricturing can cause symptoms of pyloric stenosis.

Ileal Symptoms

The terminal ileum is the classic site for Crohn's disease (Fig. 6.7a). Pain in the right iliac fossa can be the only symptom, although more often there is an alteration in bowel habit, with looseness and increased frequency. Pain is often the dominant symptom, and in contrast to ulcerative colitis, there is more pain than might be expected from the extent of the disease. This may be due to the inflammatory lesions alone, abscess formation, or intestinal obstruction due to stricture formation. Anorexia, weight loss, general lack of well-being and anaemia are common. With more extensive involvement of the small intestine, biochemical features of malabsorption supervene, although frank steatorrhoea is rare (Fig. 6.7b). Colonic involvement produces symptoms similar to ulcerative colitis although the segmental distribution of Crohn's disease is not as clear-cut. Areas of severe ulceration may be focal and interspersed with long segments of normal colon. The rectum may be normal even in the presence of severe proximal disease.

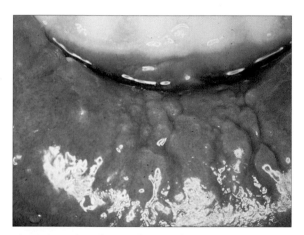

Fig. 6.5 Crohn's disease: lip irregularity.

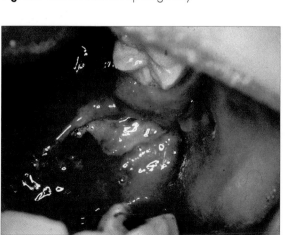

Fig. 6.6 Crohn's disease: oral ulceration.

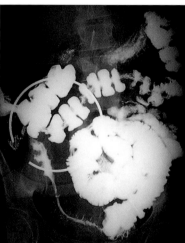

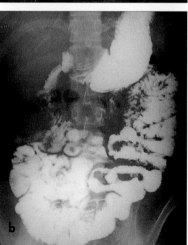

Fig. 6.7 a. Crohn's disease of the terminal ileum. **b.** extensive jejunal Crohn's disease.

Anal Symptoms

Anal lesions include skin tags (Fig. 6.8), fissuring and ulceration which is indolent and relatively painless. Anorectal fistulae are also common. Pain indicates secondary infection and perianal abscesses. The anus maybe the only area affected.

Associated Features

These can exist with either Crohn's disease or ulcerative colitis (Fig. 6.9), although the relative frequencies vary.

Eye Lesions

The most common lesions are episcleritis and iritis which present as sore, red eyes (Fig. 6.10).

Skin Lesions

Skin lesions include erythema nodosum, a red tender, raised lesion most commonly seen on the shins (Fig. 6.11). The lesions develop in sequence and

fade like a bruise. They may also be due to drug treatment with sulphasalazine. Vasculitic lesions of all severities may be seen (Fig. 6.12). Pyoderma gangrenosum is a much rarer complication characterized by necrotic ulceration which can extend rapidly (Fig. 6.13). The purulent discharge from this unpleasant lesion is sterile unless secondary infection occurs.

Joint Involvement

Seronegative arthritis or arthralgia typically involves the large joints with a predilection for knees and ankles. Effusions occur, but there is no erosive destruction of the joints (Fig. 6.14). There is also an association between ulcerative colitis and ankylosing spondylitis.

Liver Disease

Liver disease is an uncommon, but potentially serious complication. The majority of those with abnormal liver function tests have no clinically significant liver abnormality. A very small number of patients with ulcerative colitis develop sclerosing cholangitis (see Chapter 5). In some cases, the liver disease may precede the onset of colitis. Carcinoma of the bile duct is a less common, but serious, association. The development of painless obstructive jaundice in a patient with ulcerative colitis is a sinister sign.

EXAMINATION

General examination may reveal some of the associated features mentioned above. Signs of anaemia, recent weight loss and oedema from hypoproteinaemia may be noted. The abdomen may be tender over an inflamed intestine, particularly in Crohn's disease. A palpable mass is most commonly

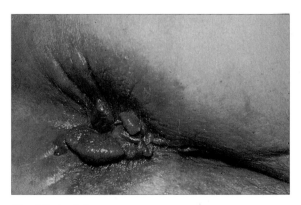

Fig. 6.8 Anal skin tags.

EXTRA-INTESTINAL MANIFESTATIONS OF INFLAMMATORY BOWEL DISEASE			
Eyes	**Skin**	**Joints**	**Liver**
iritis	erythema nodosum	arthralgia	sclerosing cholangitis
episcleritis	vasculitis	seronegative arthropathy	bile duct carcinoma
		effusions	

Fig. 6.9 Extra-intestinal manifestations of inflammatory bowel disease.

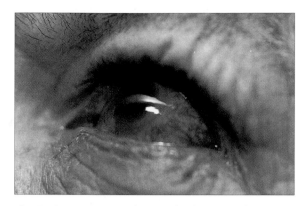

Fig. 6.10 Iritis is a complication developing in about 5% of patients with ulcerative colitis and Crohn's disease. It is not related to the severity of inflammatory bowel disease, only one third of cases being associated with an acute exacerbation.

felt in the right iliac fossa over the terminal ileum. Distension, increased borborygmi and visible peristalsis are found if small-intestinal obstruction has occurred. Colonic distension can occur to a dangerous degree without being detectable clinically.

Careful inspection of the perineum should precede rectal examination. The perianal skin in Crohn's disease has a dusky, violaceous appearance. Induration and tenderness, skin tags, abscess formation or the discharging punctum of an anorectal fistula are all highly suggestive of Crohn's disease. The perineum is usually normal in ulcerative colitis.

The anal canal is normal in ulcerative colitis, but may be irregular and ulcerated with chronic fissures in Crohn's disease. Rectal examination may not be possible because of pain. This indicates sepsis, as the tags and induration of Crohn's disease are not painful in themselves. The rectal mucosa may feel irregular, velvety or normal in both diseases.

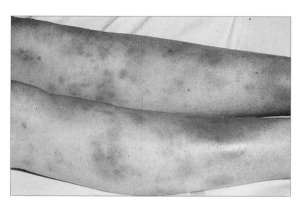

Fig. 6.11 Erythema nodosum.

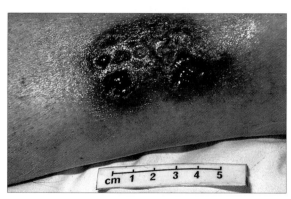

Fig. 6.13 Pyoderma gangrenosum.

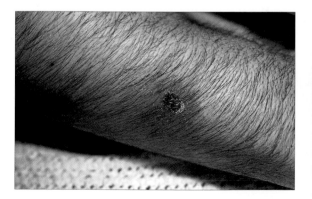

Fig. 6.12 Vasculitis.

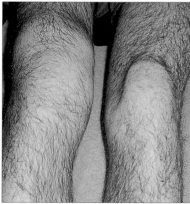

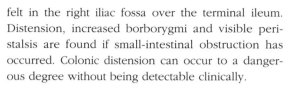

Fig. 6.14 Knee with effusion.

INVESTIGATIONS

Blood Tests

It is important to determine the haemoglobin and white cell count. Profuse diarrhoea may lead to significant electrolyte abnormalities; plasma protein and albumin levels will give an indication of the intensity of inflammation and nutritional state. A low albumin level is a poor prognostic factor in severe attacks of colitis.

Radiology

Patients with a severe attack of colitis should have a plain abdominal X-ray taken. As a badly inflamed colon will not retain stools, the extent of the colitis can be inferred from the presence or absence of faecal matter. Colonic dilatation indicates deep ulceration with an increased risk of colonic perforation. A 'megacolon' is an abnormal colon which is dilated to 6.5 cm or more (Fig. 6.15). The term 'toxic megacolon' is misleading, as the colon can dilate without

the patient being particularly unwell or clinically 'toxic'. Perforation can also occur without dilatation, however, and free air in the abdomen should be looked for in all cases. In severe colitis, the ulceration may be so extensive that only small areas of mucosa survive. The presence of these 'mucosal islands' and oedema of the colonic wall are strong indications of the need for early surgery (Fig. 6.16).

Barium enema examination will give useful information about the extent of disease in ulcerative colitis (Fig. 6.17) and the distribution of disease, which is helpful in making the diagnosis in Crohn's colitis (Fig. 6.18). This is important for the immediate treatment of the acute attack and also has long-term implications with regard to the follow-up of ulcerative colitis. In acute colitis, a barium enema performed without bowel preparation (an 'instant' enema) will give adequate information about the extent of the disease and its severity (Fig. 6.19).

When small bowel disease is suspected a barium follow-through examination, with compression techniques to demonstrate the terminal ileum, is preferred. It is important to remember that the terminal ileum may also be affected by tuberculosis (Fig. 6.20),

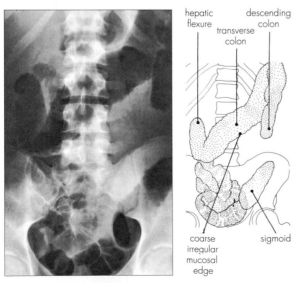

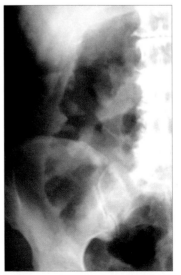

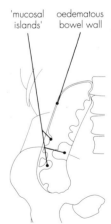

Fig. 6.15 Colonic dilatation: the transverse colon is dilated and has a coarse mucosal edge, without haustra. These changes indicate deep ulceration into the colonic muscle layer.

Fig. 6.16 Mucosal islands, oedema of the bowel wall and dilatation in ulcerative colitis.

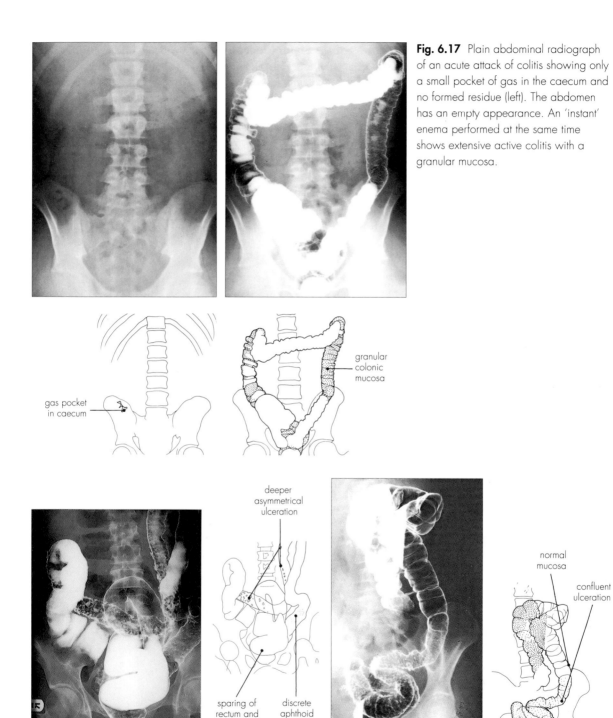

Fig. 6.17 Plain abdominal radiograph of an acute attack of colitis showing only a small pocket of gas in the caecum and no formed residue (left). The abdomen has an empty appearance. An 'instant' enema performed at the same time shows extensive active colitis with a granular mucosa.

gas pocket in caecum

granular colonic mucosa

deeper asymmetrical ulceration

normal mucosa

confluent ulceration

sparing of rectum and sigmoid colon

discrete aphthoid ulceration

Fig. 6.18 Crohn's disease involving the colon. Note the normal rectum and sigmoid loop, aphthoid ulceration in the descending colon and more severe ulceration of the transverse colon, where the disease is asymmetrical.

Fig. 6.19 'Instant' enema in acute attack of ulcerative colitis with distal ulceration. The ulcers are shallow and confluent, and there is an abrupt transition to normal mucosa in the lower descending colon.

Nuclear Medicine

Isotope techniques are useful in clinically difficult cases. A quantity of the patient's white blood cells is labelled with an isotope. The white cells migrate to areas of acute inflammation and allow localization of active intestinal disease or intra-abdominal abscesses.

TREATMENT

Treatment of ulcerative colitis and Crohn's colitis is the same and depends on the distribution of the disease.

Ulcerative Colitis

Medical
The mainstays of medical treatment are the corticosteroids hydrocortisone and prednisolone, and the various preparations of 5-aminosalicylic acid (5-ASA), sulphasalazine, mesalazine, olsalazine and balsalazide (Fig. 6.27).

PROCTITIS
Disease confined to the rectum is best treated with a topical preparation. Mild attacks will respond to prednisolone suppositories. Foam preparations of prednisolone metasulphabenzoate or hydrocortisone are effective for more severe inflammation and can be retained in the rectum when the patient is ambulatory.

Suppositories and liquid enemas which contain 5-ASA or sulphasalazine are useful alternatives.

DISTAL COLITIS
Suppositories are of little value when the upper limit of the disease cannot be seen with a rigid sigmoidoscope. Foam enemas will adequately reach the sigmoid colon, but may not be sufficient for more proximal disease. In these cases, liquid enemas which contain either prednisolone-21-phosphate or prednisolone metasulphabenzoate may be more effective. The systemic absorption through the colon is less with the metasulphabenzoate but both are equally effective. Liquid enemas should be administered on retiring at night but foam can be used by day as well (Fig. 6.28).

It is usual to combine enema treatment with oral therapy using a 5-ASA preparation such as sulphasalazine, mesalazine or olsalazine. These are all effective treatments for mild to moderate acute attacks, and for the maintenance of remission of ulcerative colitis in particular.

EXTENSIVE AND DISTAL COLITIS
Enemas cannot be relied upon to reach the transverse colon, so oral treatment is usually necessary for these patients. Mild to moderate attacks will need

TREATMENT OF ACUTE COLITIS			
	Proctitis	**Distal colitis**	**Total colitis**
Corticosteroids	suppositories foam enemas	liquid/foam enemas	oral or intravenous
5-aminosalicylates	suppositories liquid enema	liquid enema oral	oral
Sulphasalazine	suppositories	liquid enema oral	oral

Fig. 6.27 Treatment of acute colitis.

oral prednisolone, and patients should be reviewed frequently to ensure that they respond to therapy. Failure to respond to adequate doses of oral prednisolone is an indication for hospital admission.

A severe attack that requires hospital admission needs treatment with intravenous hydrocortisone or prednisolone. The routine use of various antibiotics and intravenous feeding has not been shown to improve the outcome of these patients who should be cared for by a gastroenterologist, working in close concert with surgical colleagues. Close monitoring of such patients is essential in order to identify any deterioration or complications at an early stage.

Maintenance
5-AMINOSALICYLIC ACID
It is usual to advise that maintenance treatment with a 5-ASA drug for ulcerative colitis be continued indefinitely to reduce the chances of disease relapse. With treatment, approximately 80% of patients will remain in remission whereas, without it, up to 80% will experience a relapse within a year. Common side effects of sulphasalazine include headache, anorexia and nausea, and skin rashes, some of which may be reduced by the use of enteric-coated tablets. Male infertility is not infrequent, but is reversible if treatment is stopped. Less common but more severe side effects include photosensitivity reactions and blood dyscrasia. Mesalazine, olsalazine and balsalazide have been developed with the intention of avoiding these side effects, which are due mainly to the sulphapyridine part of the molecule. In this they have been successful, and male infertility can be avoided. Some patients still have a reaction to salicylate, and both mesalazine and olsalazine preparations have been reported to cause diarrhoea in a small number of patients. There have also been sporadic reports of nephrotoxicity with mesalazine.

CORTICOSTEROIDS
Corticosteroids are not suitable for routine maintenance therapy because of their predictable, dose-related side effects. When remissions are short-lived despite 5-ASA treatment, some patients may be maintained on low doses of prednisolone given on alternate days. This dosage regimen appears to avoid many of the expected steroid side effects.

When the patient is dependent on steroids to maintain a remission, the immunosuppressive action of azathioprine may be helpful. In some cases, the steroids can then be stopped and remission maintained. Azathioprine may cause an influenza-like illness within three weeks of starting treatment. In the long term, there is a risk of marrow suppression which can affect all blood cell series. For this reason it is imperative that those receiving azathioprine have their haemoglobin, white cell and platelet counts regularly checked, every six to eight weeks, for as long as treatment continues. Marrow suppression is rare, and reversible, but potentially extremely serious.

ANTIDIARRHOEAL DRUGS
Symptomatic treatment with antidiarrhoeal drugs can be of great benefit, but they should be used with caution in an acute relapse. Antidiarrhoeal therapy can exacerbate the proximal constipation which occurs in acute distal colitis. The right colon becomes loaded with stool and laxatives are often needed to overcome this problem. Constipation is a common cause of some of the pain experienced by those with colitis. In more extensive, severe disease, antidiarrhoeal drugs may contribute to colonic stasis and dilatation.

For a summary of the possible side effects caused by maintenance treatment, see Fig. 6.29.

SELF-ADMINISTRATION OF A FOAM ENEMA

1. shake the container before use

2. the easiest way is to stand with one foot raised on a chair

3. gently insert the nozzle into the rectum

4. inject the foam

Fig. 6.28 Administration of foam enemas.

SIDE EFFECTS OF DRUGS USED IN COLITIS		
Steroids	**Sulphasalazine/5-ASA**	**Azathioprine**
moon-face	headache	
hirsutism	nausea	nausea/abdominal pain
trunkal obesity	skin rashes	influenza-like illness
acne	diarrhoea (MO)	
diabetes mellitus	nephrotoxicity (M?)	
adrenal suppression	photosensitivity (S)	
osteoporosis	blood dyscrasias (S)	marrow suppression
S = sulphasalazine M = mesalazine O = olsalazine		

Fig. 6.29 Side effects of drugs used in colitis.

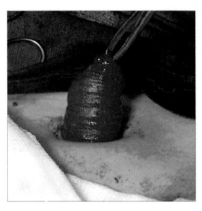

Fig. 6.30 A healthy Brooke ileostomy.

Surgery

Surgery is an integral part of the treatment of inflammatory bowel disease and offers a cure for ulcerative colitis. It is relatively easy to decide on the need for surgery in the case of severe colitis which has not responded to optimal medical treatment, although the exact timing may still cause difficulty. It is much more difficult for those patients whose disease runs a relapsing course with reasonable health between attacks, and for those who have chronically active disease and who seldom feel completely well. Most patients are reluctant to consider surgery. There is understandable fear about the procedure and there is an overpowering desire to avoid an ileostomy. As a result, many patients continue to tolerate sub-optimal levels of health with intermittent symptoms and continuous medication. It behoves the doctor to consider surgery not as a last resort when all else fails, but as one of several therapeutic options available to him and his patients.

The decision to submit the patient to surgery should be taken after adequate discussion amongst the physician, surgeon, patient and their family, with the support of specialist nursing staff, such as stomatherapists. It is sometimes helpful to a patient to meet someone who has undergone similar surgery, has a stoma, and who is now well (Fig. 6.30). Organizations such as the National Association for Colitis and Crohn's Disease (in the UK) are a useful source of information and support for patients and their families.

PANPROCTOCOLECTOMY

The standard elective operation for ulcerative colitis is panproctocolectomy. This involves removing the entire colon and rectum (Fig. 6.31a), and forming a permanent ileostomy (Fig. 6.31b). An alternative is to leave the rectum *in situ* with the proximal end either brought to the skin as a mucous fistula, or over-sewn and left in the pelvis, and to perform colectomy and ileostomy (Fig. 6.31c). This procedure has a lower morbidity rate for patients who require emergency surgery. It leaves the possibility of restoring intestinal continuity with the formation of either an ileorectal anastomosis or an ileal pouch. An ileorectal anastomosis (Fig. 6.31d) is well suited to Crohn's disease when the rectum is spared, but in ulcerative colitis there remains the problem of disease relapse and the long-term cancer risk in the retained rectum.

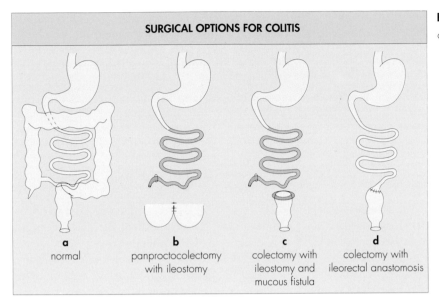

SURGICAL OPTIONS FOR COLITIS

a
normal

b
panproctocolectomy
with ileostomy

c
colectomy with
ileostomy and
mucous fistula

d
colectomy with
ileorectal anastomosis

Fig. 6.31 Surgical options for colitis

In restorative proctocolectomy, a reservoir or 'pouch' is fashioned from the terminal ileum. This is then anastomosed to the anal sphincters after the removal of the rectum. A covering loop ileostomy is required temporarily and is usually closed after approximately three months (Fig. 6.32). This operation is not suitable for Crohn's disease because of the possibility of subsequent small intestinal disease affecting the reservoir, which might have to be removed with the loss of a substantial amount of small intestine.

COLON CANCER AND ULCERATIVE COLITIS

Ulcerative colitis is associated with an increased risk of colon cancer. It is greatest for those who have had ulcerative colitis for more than 8 years, and whose disease is extensive or total. The risk rises with the duration of the disease, and the risk has been estimated as being between 5 and 17 times greater than that in the normal population. For this reason, patients with extensive colitis should have a regular surveillance colonoscopy examination every other year. During these examinations, a careful search is made for macroscopic lesions, and multiple biopsies are obtained to look for dysplastic change. Severe dysplasia in a macroscopic lesion carries a high risk of cancer elsewhere in the colon and is a strong indication of the need for elective colectomy.

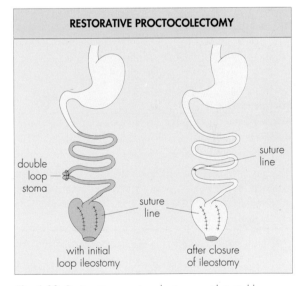

RESTORATIVE PROCTOCOLECTOMY

double
loop
stoma

suture
line

suture
line

with initial
loop ileostomy

after closure
of ileostomy

Fig. 6.32 Restorative proctocolectomy: with initial loop ileostomy, and after closure of ileostomy.

Crohn's Disease

The treatment of Crohn's disease affecting the colon (Crohn's colitis) is the same as for ulcerative colitis. Treatment of Crohn's disease of the small intestine depends upon the distribution of the disease and the symptoms caused. For example, a localized lesion in the terminal ileum will require oral prednisolone in a dose similar to that used for colitis, and for a similar duration.

Medical

The addition of antibiotics such as metronidazole and ampicillin is sometimes worthwhile. Evidence that the response to treatment with antibiotics and steroids is any better than the response to steroids alone, is lacking. They are best used when there is concern that secondary infection is playing a signficiant part in the patient's symptoms.

The 5-ASA drugs are designed to release the active drug into the colon, so their effectiveness in small intestinal disease is limited. A new preparation which acts in the small bowel is undergoing study.

The antidiarrhoeal drugs codeine, loperamide and diphenoxylate are useful for symptom control as are antispasmodics such as mebeverine and dicyclomine. Cholestyramine (an ion-exchange resin which binds bile acids in the intestine) can reduce diarrhoea when it is caused by excess bile acids entering the colon in cases of ileal dysfunction and after ileal resection.

Maintenance

Maintenance therapy for Crohn's disease of the small intestine is generally unsatisfactory, unlike that for ulcerative colitis and, to a lesser extent, Crohn's colitis. If relapses are frequent, or when satisfactory symptom control can only be achieved by continuous use of steroids, azathioprine can be used as an immunosuppressant.

Diet

Many patients recognize that there are certain foods which exacerbate their symptoms, and that these should be avoided. When the intestine is severely strictured, pain, distension and nausea may be caused by partial obstruction. Avoidance of foods which resist mechanical breakdown, such as meat, fruits like oranges, raisins and dates, stalks of fibrous vegetables, and peanuts, is worthwhile. Any calorie deficit can be made up by using liquid food supplements.

Great interest has been generated by the use of elemental diets as primary, rather than nutritional, therapy in Crohn's disease. These diets contain proteins, carbohydrates and fats in predigested forms and are thought to act by removing any antigenic stimulus to the disease. Studies have shown these diets to be as effective as prednisolone when treatment of an acute attack has to be continued for several weeks, but there is no long-term benefit with regard to relapse rates. A new study has demonstrated that non-elemental liquid diets may be as effective as an elemental preparation in producing remission in acute Crohn's disease.

For those few patients whose intestine is no longer able to function adequately, parenteral nutrition is valuable. It is most commonly used for those with extensive small-intestinal disease during an acute attack or in the perioperative period. In extreme cases, often after repeated intestinal resections, parenteral nutrition can be continued at home. This requires expert monitoring by a specialist gastroenterology unit.

A large trial which compared a high residue, low refined carbohdyrate diet with a more traditional British diet, rich in refined carbohydrate and low in fibre, showed no difference in the incidence of relapse, complications or surgery in patients with Crohn's disease.

Surgery

Crohn's disease, unlike ulcerative colitis, cannot be cured by surgery, but the judicious use of limited intervention can be dramatically effective. After resection of the diseased terminal ileum with ileocolic anastomosis, 50% of patients will be free of disease 5 years later. This should be borne in mind when long-term use of potentially harmful drugs is necessary to maintain reasonably good health.

For those with stricturing disease at one or more sites, the procedure of strictureplasty is useful. The distorted intestine is refashioned to deal with obstructive symptoms but is not resected. The disease may become quiescent and so useful intestinal function can be conserved. The long-term outcome of such surgery has proved to be surprisingly good, considering that the diseased bowel remains in situ.

Pouch operations are not suitable for Crohn's disease. A variety of limited surgical procedures are often needed to deal with complications such as abscesses, fistula formation (both internal and external), and localized anal disease.

POINTS TO REMEMBER

Ulcerative colitis

- Affects only the colon
- Typically has a relapsing course
- Can be cured by surgery
- Is potentially fatal in a severe acute attack
- May be complicated by colonic dilatation when severe
- Carries an increased risk of colon cancer in extensive or total colitis of 8 years duration or more

Crohn's disease

- Can affect any part of the gastrointestinal tract
- Cannot be cured by surgery
- Is an important cause of growth retardation in children and adolescents
- Does not carry the same cancer risk as ulcerative colitis

7. Functional (Dysmotility) Disorders of the Bowel

INTRODUCTION

Up to 10% of all consultations with general practitioners relate to symptoms from the gastrointestinal tract. Approximately half the patients will be dyspeptic and about a third of the remainder will have symptoms referable to the lower bowel.

One of the main problems for general practitioners is identifying within this enormous mass of patients the small numbers with serious and progressive bowel disease. This chapter concentrates on non-ulcer dyspepsia and irritable bowel syndrome and aims to provide useful guidelines for the clinical diagnosis of these problems, which will obviate the requirement for invasive investigations and consultant advice.

DYSPEPSIA

Following the deliberations of various working parties over the past few years, dyspepsia can now be conveniently divided on a clinical basis into four different categories (Fig. 7.1).

DIAGNOSIS

Symptoms of dysmotility type dyspepsia

- Nausea (particularly in the mornings)
- Flatulence
- Early satiety
- Upper abdominal bloating after meals
- Epigastric soreness

Clinical recognition of dyspepsia in the diagnosis of the patient who presents with heartburn and/or waterbrash, which may be exacerbated by postural changes or by various foods (see Chapter 1), is usually straightforward. Similarly, the diagnosis of patients with epigastric pain, which may or may not radiate through to the back, be eased by food, be exacerbated by hunger, be worse at night or be relieved by antacids or H_2-receptor antagonists, is also simple. Although these particular groups of patients may have no abnormalities apparent on investigation, they do respond to standard therapy with antacids and/or H_2-receptor antagonists.

The more difficult groups, which have previously been labelled functional dyspepsia but may be better referred to as dysmotility type dyspepsia, have a wide variety of symptoms which are difficult to categorize. Indeed, dysmotility type dyspepsia is probably a form of a widespread, diffuse abnormality of coordination of the gastrointestinal tract, which as yet defies categorization. The aetiology is poorly understood and therefore treatment is less than satisfactory.

INVESTIGATION AND MANAGEMENT

Almost invariably, investigations in patients with dysmotility type dyspepsia are unremarkable and although a large proportion of them will be infected with *Helicobacter pylori*, there is as yet no evidence

CLINICAL VARIATIONS OF DYSPEPSIA
reflux-like dyspepsia
ulcer-like dyspepsia
dysmotility type dyspepsia
aerophagia and idiopathic dyspepsia

Fig. 7.1 Clinical variations of dyspepsia.

that eradicating the organism relieves the symptoms. Until recently it was thought that patients in this group had more than average levels of stress, anxiety and psychoneurotic disorders, but this is not borne out by prospective studies or by clinical practice.

More sophisticated tests have revealed that more than 50% have abnormalities of gastric emptying, with abnormal motor complexes in the antrum of the stomach in particular and also with reflux of gastric contents into the oesophagus. These symptoms tend to be refractory to standard forms of therapy and investigations are usually fruitless. Symptomatic treatment with anti-emetics such as metoclopramide or domperidone may relieve nausea, and more recently the use of cisapride, a cholinergic prokinetic drug, has been of some benefit. Usually all that can be offered to patients is careful explanation and reassurance, often after endoscopy. Dietary manipulation may occasionally be helpful, particularly the withdrawal of dairy foods and/or wheat- based foods, in a manner similar to that used for the management of irritable bowel syndrome.

Another probable form of dysmotility dyspepsia is the condition of compulsive air swallowing (aerophagia), which is fortunately rare but can be very disabling for patients. Management of this condition is extremely difficult, and occasionally sedation with chlorpromazine and/or nasogastric intubation is required to break the cycle of air swallowing. Patients often have evidence of other compulsive forms of behaviour.

One of the difficulties arising in the clinical management of dysmotility type dyspepsia is selecting those patients who would benefit from further investigation. The British Society of Gastroenterology recommendations for a common-sense basis for management of this condition are shown in Fig. 7.2.

Guidelines for Treatment of Dysmotility Type Dyspepsia

The mainstay of management is a careful history, examination and positive diagnosis, with an explanation to the patient of the possible source of the symptoms and reassurance that the condition is likely to be self-limiting. It is also important that patients understand that there is no easy remedy for the problem, and a variety of medications may need to be tried before symptom relief is obtained. Attention to diet and possible precipitating factors, such as those related to stresses in the family or at work, recent bereavement or moving house, may be useful, and withdrawal of triggering factors is obviously of great importance. Unfortunately, after some months of reassurance and attempts at treatment, patients may demand referral for further investigations and this pressure may be difficult to resist. In these circumstances, an open access endoscopy is probably the most appropriate form of investigation, but is usually unhelpful. There is certainly no indication for treatment with the more potent acid suppressants and/or anti-helicobacter therapy until this has been shown to relieve the symptoms of dysmotility type dyspepsia.

POINTS TO REMEMBER

- Endoscopy is not necessary if a 'normal' barium meal has already been performed
- It is pointless prescribing H_2-receptor antagonists in patients who continue to abuse tobacco and/or alcohol

---

RECOMMENDATIONS FOR THE MANAGEMENT OF DYSPEPSIA

Require early investigation
aged over 45 with new dyspepsia
symptoms recur after adequate therapy
recurrent symptoms in a patient with known gastric ulcer
presence of dysphagia, weight loss, bleeding, vomiting, anaemia

Do not require investigation
age less than 45
known duodenal ulcer
no trial of antacids
no trial of H_2-receptor antagonists
typical reflux symptoms
symptoms suggestive of irritable bowel syndrome

Fig. 7.2 Recommendations for the management of dyspepsia.

IRRITABLE BOWEL SYNDROME

The aetiology of the ubiquitous irritable bowel syndrome (IBS) remains obscure. There is now good evidence to show that patients with IBS may have abnormalities of motor contraction of the intestine anywhere from the oesophagus to the rectum. Although symptoms may be focused on the lower bowel, careful history taking will often reveal dysmotility type dyspeptic symptoms as well. Previous studies have shown that some of the most debilitating IBS symptoms, such as abdominal distention after meals and lower abdominal pain, may emanate from the small intestine. The causes of the patchy distribution of the condition remain unknown.

DIAGNOSIS

Symptoms

- Alternating constipation and diarrhoea
- Excessive rectal mucus production
- Marked flatulence
- Lower abdominal distention
- Colicky abdominal pain

Classically patients present with one or more of the symptoms given above. The combination of two or more of these symptoms (the so-called Manning criteria), may lead to a positive diagnosis of IBS, obviating the requirement for invasive investigation. Although the aetiology is obscure, there is no doubt that patients with IBS may exhibit incoordinate contractions of the bowel in response to external stresses. These may be psychological or physical stresses, such as emotion or, in the clinic, insertion of a hand into cold water. The abnormal contractility of the bowel may be manifested in any part of the colon and/or the small intestine and may not necessarily relate to the severity of the patient's symptoms.

The precipitating factors which are commonly recognized to be associated with irritable bowel syndrome are shown in Fig. 7.3. There is often a history in childhood or teenage years of abdominal symptoms, perhaps exacerbated by inappropriate use of purgatives to ensure a regular bowel habit.

Symptom Complexes

The condition appears to be more common in women than men and may be exacerbated just before the onset of the menstrual period. Classically, lower abdominal distention occurs, worsening during the day and at its worst in the evening. This may or may not be associated with marked flatulence and is partially relieved by defaecation. These patients tend to visit the bathroom several times early in the morning, often associated with tenesmus and the passage of excessive amounts of mucus. They feel exhausted after their frequent trips to the bathroom and may even feel faint. The stools do not contain blood, and there should be no associated weight loss or vomiting.

The other variant of the syndrome is characterized by bouts of abdominal pain which is usually colicky in nature, often associated with constipation, and the pain is usually relieved by defaecation. The pain can occur anywhere in the abdomen but most commonly in the left iliac fossa or suprapubic, and it may be

FACTORS ASSOCIATED WITH IRRITABLE BOWEL SYNDROME
stress (psychological/physical)
neuroticism
poor eating habit
beverages
female

Fig. 7.3 Precipitating factors commonly associated with irritable bowel syndrome.

INDICATIONS FOR REFERRAL OF IBS PATIENTS
rectal bleeding
weight loss
persistent vomiting
evidence of systemic disease such as joint disease, eye disease or skin disease

Fig. 7.4 Patients with irritable bowel syndrome should be referred for further investigation if any of these symptoms are present.

exacerbated in women by sexual intercourse or the menstrual period. Often such patients are referred initially to gynaecologists and are then sent on to gastroenterologists once gynaecological investigations have been completed and have been found to show no abnormality.

INVESTIGATIONS

As most patients are generally healthy and relatively young, finding that the characteristic symptoms are present means that no further investigations (flexible sigmoidoscopy and barium enema) are indicated. Patients should be referred for investigations where weight loss and/or rectal bleeding are present, or where the symptoms prove refractory to the usual management approaches (Fig. 7.4.).

MANAGEMENT

Although numerous trials have been conducted for the various medications that are offered for patients with IBS, it is clear that there is no one specific ther-

apy or combination of therapies that can be relied upon to produce a marked improvement in symptoms for the majority of patients.

The cornerstone of management remains explanation and reassurance. Simply telling the patient there is nothing wrong with them and sending them away with a prescription for an antispasmodic or similar medication is of little value and almost inevitably results in a poor response. The most effective form of management is to spend some time with the patient, clearly explaining what is known about the causes of IBS and the various treatment options available.

Often simple explanation is enough to allow patients to accept that their symptoms are not representative of serious organic disease and that the whole episode should be self-limiting. When this approach fails medical treatment may be offered, as described below (Fig. 7.5).

If the symptoms of constipation are predominant, a high-fibre diet, preferably provided by dietary modification rather than medication, is advised. In patients in whom colicky pain and diarrhoea are more prominent, antispasmodics (mebeverine, peppermint oil) may be tried but are recommended only for short periods.

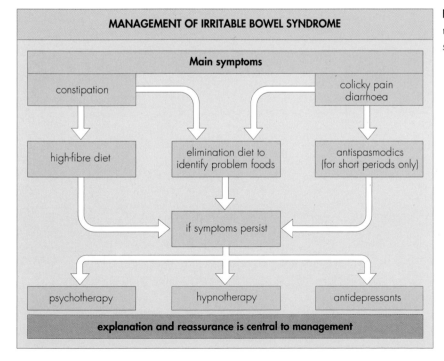

Fig. 7.5 The approach to management of irritable bowel syndrome.

A dietary approach may be helpful, in particular there is some evidence that an elimination diet, with patients taking just meat, fruit, fish and vegetables for a short period, is of value. This approach also allows the patient to take control of their symptoms and may also identify various foods or beverages to which they are intolerant.

Usually a combination of the two approaches above is successful in the majority of patients but there are some unfortunate sufferers of IBS whose symptoms are protracted and may even lead to admission to hospital. In these cases, a psychotherapeutic approach may be necessary, and even hypnotherapy has been shown to be of value. A trial of antidepressants may be warranted and is often surprisingly successful.

The wrong approach to patients with IBS is for them to be briefly examined, have a brisk sigmoidoscopy, be sent for a barium enema and told that the results of the investigations are normal and there is nothing wrong with them. Hopefully this form of treatment is becoming outmoded; and the great majority of patients with IBS should be managed in general practice.

POINTS TO REMEMBER

- A positive diagnosis of IBS should be made
- IBS is a self-limiting disease
- Prominent gynaecological symptoms require investigation

8. Colorectal Cancer and Polyps

INTRODUCTION

Colorectal cancer is a common and important cause of death and morbidity in the United Kingdom. Some 27,000 new cases occur each year, with an annual death toll of approximately 20,000. Of those who develop colorectal cancer, 25% are less than 60 years old at the time of presentation. In the UK, only bronchial carcinoma is commoner.

Colonic cancer in particular often presents late in its development with the result that many patients have advanced disease, either locally or with disseminated metastases, by the time they experience significant symptoms. Early detection depends on a high index of clinical suspicion, followed by prompt and complete investigation of suspicious symptoms.

Pathogenesis

Environment

There is a geographical variation in the incidence of colorectal cancer which indicates that environmental factors play a part in the aetiology.

Diet

Conflicting views exist about the role of diet. It has been postulated by some that a diet containing high quantities of fat and a dearth of dietary fibre may be associated with an increased risk of colorectal tumours, but this is refuted by others. The hypothesis that high bile acid levels act as a co-carcinogen, and that slower transit, due to low dietary fibre content, allows a greater time for dietary carcinogens to be in contact with gut mucosa, seeks to explain the high incidence of colorectal cancer in western society, but the case remains unproven.

Genetics

A genetic susceptibility plays a part in some cases of colorectal cancer. In familial adenomatous polyposis (previously polyposis coli; Fig. 8.1) the condition is transmitted as an autosomal dominant with high penetration. People with this condition will all develop colonic carcinoma in time. Various family cancer syndromes have been identified. There is an increased risk to those individuals who have a first degree relation (sibling, parent or offspring) with colorectal cancer, and the relative risk increases with the number of cases in the family.

High Risk Conditions

Colonic adenomas, which occur sporadically in the population, confer an increased risk of subsequent cancer. Ulcerative colitis, which involves all or a substantial proportion of the colon, is associated with an increased risk of colorectal cancer. This becomes significant after the colitis has been present for 8 years.

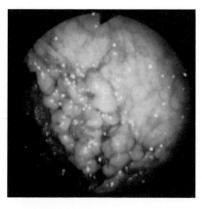

Fig. 8.1 Familial adenomatous polyposis. A conglomerate of innumerable small polyps covers the colon wall like a carpet. This is the most common presentation.

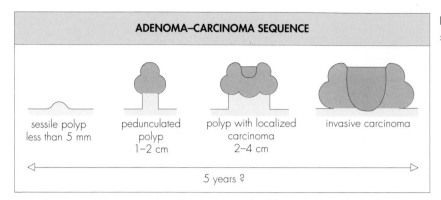

Fig. 8.2 Adenoma–carcinoma sequence.

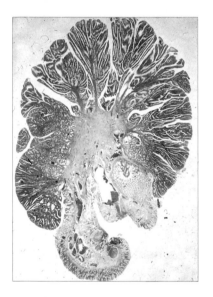 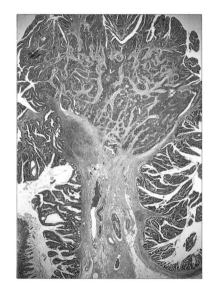

Fig. 8.3 Histological appearances demonstrating the difference between benign and malignant adenomatous lesions. In the benign case (left), the muscularis is intact, whereas in the malignant lesion (right), the muscularis mucosa is obviously invaded by malignant epithelium. Malignant glands in the lymphatics are seen close to the base of the stalk. H & E stain.

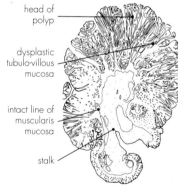 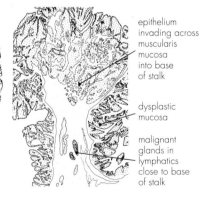

AETIOLOGY

Most colonic cancers probably arise in an area of mucosa which has initially undergone benign adenomatous change, and which has subsequently become malignant. The adenoma–carcinoma sequence is shown in Figs 8.2 and 8.3. The time-scale for this transformation is thought to be approximately 5 years.

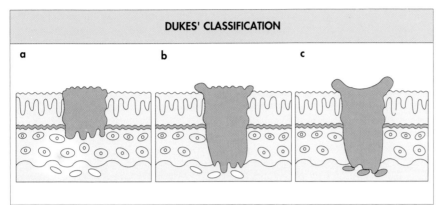

Fig. 8.4 Dukes' classification of colorectal cancer. **a.** The tumour has not penetrated the bowel wall. **b.** The bowel has been penetrated but the lymph nodes are not involved. **c.** The lymph nodes have been invaded by the tumour.

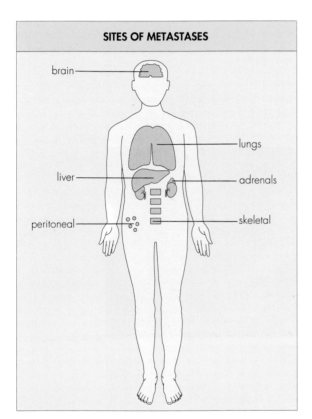

Fig. 8.5 The sites of metastasis in colorectal cancer. The liver and lungs are most commonly affected.

PROGNOSIS

Colorectal cancer is a curable disease with 5-year survival figures being closely linked to the extent of the tumour at the time of surgical treatment, as determined using Dukes' classification (Fig. 8.4). Over the past 20 years or so, however, the 5-year survival rates have not improved significantly. As with many other conditions, this reflects the fact that improvements in operative and anaesthetic techniques are probably being offset by the perioperative morbidity incurred by an older population. In addition, there remains the problem that colorectal cancer, and colonic tumours in particular, often do not cause significant symptoms until the tumour is locally extensive or has already metastasized, most commonly to the liver and lungs (Fig. 8.5). Bone, brain, peritoneal and adrenal metastases occur less frequently.

DIAGNOSIS

Symptoms

Rectal	*Left-sided*	*Right-sided*
• Bleeding	• Bleeding	• Anaemia
• Mucus	• Mucus	• Diarrhoea
• Wet wind	• Altered	• Abdominal
• Tenesmus	bowels	pain
• Incomplete	• Constipation/	• Malaise/
evacuation	diarrhoea	weight loss
• Rectal pain	• Abdominal	• Mass in
• Rectal mass	pain	abdomen
	• Increased	
	noise	
	• Malaise/	
	weight loss	
	• Mass in	
	abdomen	

Colonic and rectal carcinoma (Figs 8.6 and 8.7) can present with any of a wide range of symptoms. Rectal cancer commonly presents with rectal bleeding, often accompanied by mucous discharge, tenesmus and a feeling of incomplete evacuation.

Bleeding is often ignored by the patient, from fear of the diagnosis, or it is attributed to 'piles'. Alteration of bowel habit in an older person, often with alternating bouts of relative constipation and bowel looseness, suggests partial colonic obstruction, most commonly from a left-sided lesion. Similar symptoms may be attributed to diverticular disease and this can lead to a delay in diagnosis. Others may present without bowel symptoms but may complain of fatigue and dyspnoea due to the insidious development of iron deficiency anaemia. For differential diagnosis of colonic and rectal cancer see Fig. 8.8.

EXAMINATION

When a history is obtained which suggests the diagnosis of colorectal cancer, abdominal examination is concerned with finding areas of tenderness, mass lesions, and the presence of liver enlargement. Rectal examination is mandatory. Rigid sigmoidoscopy, performed without bowel preparation, may give invaluable information and should be carried out in patients with rectal bleeding before resorting to a barium enema. If a lesion is confirmed, then tissue can be obtained for histology. Even if no tumour is seen, however, the presence of blood either on the stool, or coming from above, is an important finding and indicates the presence of a more proximal lesion.

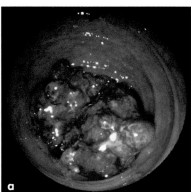

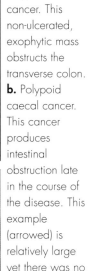

Fig. 8.6 a. Polypoid colon cancer. This non-ulcerated, exophytic mass obstructs the transverse colon. **b.** Polypoid caecal cancer. This cancer produces intestinal obstruction late in the course of the disease. This example (arrowed) is relatively large yet there was no obstruction to retrograde filling of the ileum and no dilatation of the small intestine.

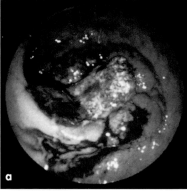

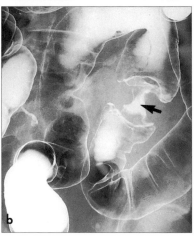

Fig. 8.7 a. Ulcerated rectal cancer. This large excavated bleeding cancer was found in the mid-rectum. **b.** 'Applecore' cancer in the distal sigmoid colon (arrowed).

DIFFERENTIAL DIAGNOSIS		
Rectal	**Left-sided**	**Right-sided**
piles	diverticular disease	appendicitis
fissure		
proctitis	colitis	Crohn's disease
	inflammatory	ileum
	infective	caecum
	ischaemic	
solitary ulcer		tuberculosis
polyp	polyp	polyp
irritable bowel	irritable bowel	irritable bowel

Fig. 8.8 Differential diagnosis of colorectal cancer.

INVESTIGATION

Barium enema is still the most easily available hospital-based investigation and high quality, double contrast films should be routinely available. Despite this technique, there are still areas of the colon which are difficult to examine fully. The sigmoid loop is notoriously difficult to demonstrate, particularly when it is affected by diverticular disease (Fig. 8.9), and the caecum may be poorly seen if the bowel preparation has been less than perfect.

When patients present with rectal bleeding, anorectal examination may be normal and a barium enema may demonstrate no lesion or only diverticular disease. In such cases, either colonoscopy or flexible sigmoidoscopy should be performed. A high yield of polyps or cancer can be expected in such patients.

Colonoscopy and flexible sigmoidoscopy differ only in extent of examination and bowel preparation

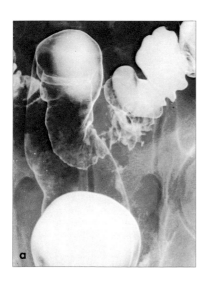

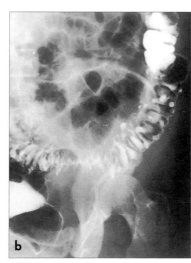

Fig. 8.9 a. Colon cancer in diverticular disease. Note the shouldering at the edge and surface irregularity of the tumour with loss of diverticula.
b. Diverticular disease. Thickened muscle is compressing the necks of the diverticula and the redundant mucosa is restricting the lumen.

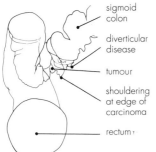

sigmoid colon
diverticular disease
tumour
shouldering at edge of carcinoma
rectum

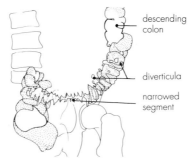

descending colon
diverticula
narrowed segment

used (Fig. 8.10). An experienced colonoscopist will take between 15 and 30 minutes to examine the entire colon in 90% of cases. Flexible sigmoidoscopy is used to view the left colon from rectum to splenic flexure and is thus an excellent way of checking a suspect sigmoid colon. It is, however, easy for inexperienced operators to overestimate the extent of their examination because of the tendency of the sigmoid colon to form loops.

Whether the instrument used is a rigid or flexible sigmoidoscope, or a colonoscope, the aim is to view the lesion and to obtain adequate tissue for histology to confirm the clinical diagnosis.

TREATMENT

Surgery remains the only curative treatment for colorectal cancer. The chances of cure depend most critically on the stage of the tumour at the time of resection and the skill of the individual surgeon. Patients with colonic tumours who undergo elective surgery will seldom require a colostomy, and new stapling techniques have increased the number of rectal tumours which can be resected without resort to a stoma. For the lowest rectal tumours, abdomino-perineal resection necessitates a permanent colostomy. Radiotherapy does not improve survival rates, but the incidence of local recurrence of rectal tumours may be reduced by perioperative radiotherapy. Adjuvant chemotherapy, with 5-fluorouracil and levamisole or folinic acid, can improve the outlook for patients with advanced local disease at the time of resection. Liver metastases may respond to chemotherapy or, in carefully selected cases, resection of a single lobe of liver with one or two isolated metastases may be worthwhile. Palliative radiotherapy, or tumour ablation using laser therapy, can be offered to patients with unresectable invasive rectal tumours.

POLYPS

A polyp is the term used for any raised growth that projects into the lumen of the intestine. In the colon, polyps may be of several histological types the most important of which is the adenoma because of its malignant potential. Detection rates have increased greatly in recent years due to the improvement in radiological techniques. Also fibre optic colonoscopy has revolutionized the treatment as it enables polyps to be removed without recourse to surgery. It is not possible to distinguish between the different types of polyps macroscopically, so all must be removed and specimens obtained for histology.

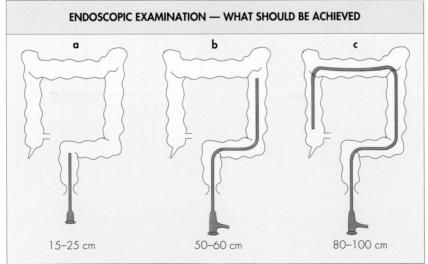

ENDOSCOPIC EXAMINATION — WHAT SHOULD BE ACHIEVED

a

b

c

15–25 cm

50–60 cm

80–100 cm

Fig. 8.10 Endoscopic examination. **a.** Rigid sigmoidoscopy: rectum, rectosigmoid.
b. Flexible sigmoidoscopy: descending colon, possibly past splenic flexure.
c. Colonoscopy: whole colon to caecum and terminal ileum, if necessary.

Metaplastic Polyps

These are the most common colonic polyps. It has been estimated that 75% of individuals over 40 years of age have at least one metaplastic polyp. These polyps are usually small, pale and sessile, and are most commonly found in the left colon (Figs 8.11 and 8.12). They have no malignant potential.

Postinflammatory Polyps

These are commonly seen in patients with inflammatory bowel disease. They occur after recovery from an acute attack of ulcerative colitis. Their presence indicates healing after severe ulceration, and their heterogeneous appearance reflects this. Many are small, reddened or pink, and irregularly shaped or worm-like. Others may be larger, firm with a white cap, and over a centimetre in diameter. They have no malignant potential, unlike the dysplasia which may develop in raised areas of colonic mucosa.

Hamartomatous Polyps

Hamartomas are non-neoplastic tumours with no malignant potential. They consist of an abnormal mixture of different tissues. The polyps of Peutz-Jeghers syndrome and juvenile polyps are of this type (see Fig. 8.13).

Peutz-Jeghers polyps are most frequently found in the small intestine. There is associated buccal and circum-oral pigmentation. There is an increased incidence of carcinomatous change in the intestinal lining adjacent to these polyps, particularly in the stomach and duodenum.

Adenomatous Polyps

Adenomas form the most important group of polyps because of their maligant potential. The majority of colonic carcinomas are thought to develop through the adenoma–carcinoma sequence, a process which may take 5 years or more. This being so, the ability to remove adenomas before maligant transformation

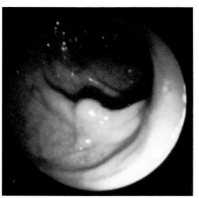

Fig. 8.11 Small metaplastic polyp on top of a mucosal fold.

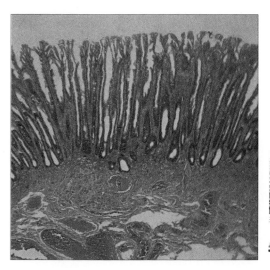

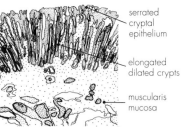

serrated cryptal epithelium

elongated dilated crypts

muscularis mucosa

Fig. 8.12 Histology of a metaplastic polyp, showing its sessile nature and the dilated crypts, which have a serrated appearance due to the uneven height of the lining cells. H & E stain, x 20.

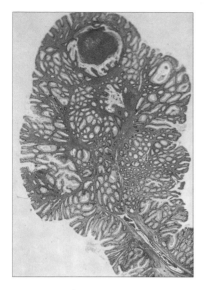
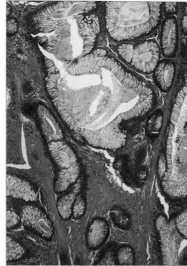

Fig. 8.13 Histology of a hamartomatous polyp. At low power (left, x12), the characteristic intermingling of glands and muscularis is seen. At high power (right, x50), the features are more obvious. There is no dysplastic element. H & E stain.

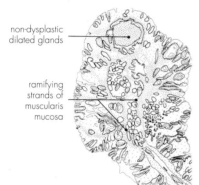

non-dysplastic dilated glands

ramifying strands of muscularis mucosa

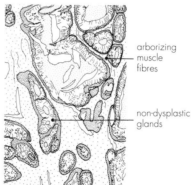

arborizing muscle fibres

non-dysplastic glands

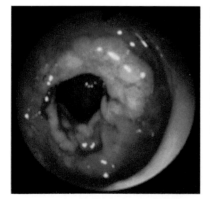

Fig. 8.14 Small, circumferential, villous adenoma. The surface of the lesion consists of multiple tiny nodules.

RISKS OF CARCINOMA IN A POLYP	
Higher	**Lower**
villous diameter greater than 2 cm	tubular diameter less than 1 cm

Fig. 8.15 Risks of carcinoma in a polyp.

could theroretically lead to a reduction in the incidence of colon cancer. This is the rationale behind follow-up programmes for patients who have adenomas.

The maligant potential of any adenoma is dependent on a number of factors. Villous adenomas (Fig. 8.14) are the most likely to develop malignant areas. They are usually pale, fleshy tumours which may secrete enough mucus to cause diarrhoea and hypokalaemia. Tubular adenomas have the lowest

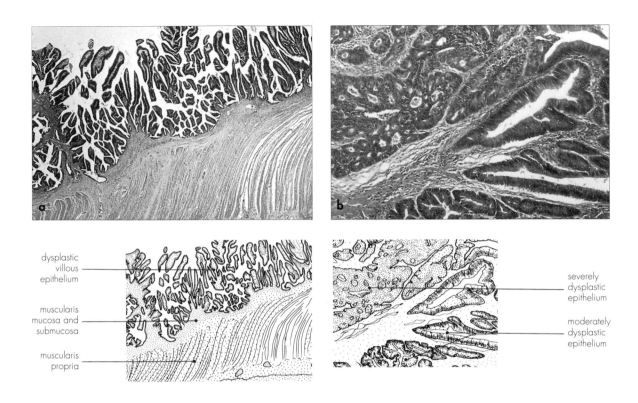

Fig. 8.16 Histology of **a** a villous (x 12), and **b** a tubular adenoma (x 75) H & E stain.

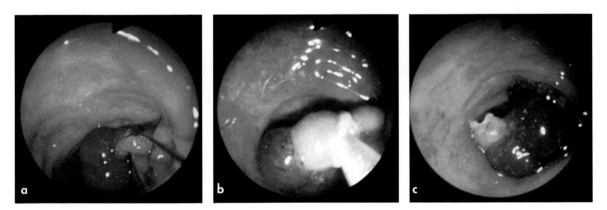

Fig. 8.17 Polypectomy of a pedunculated polyp. **a.** A snare wire is manoeuvred around the stalk. **b.** Oedematous swelling is evident at the transection line. **c.** Released polyp lies in the lumen.

potential for malignant change (Fig. 8.15). Tubulo-villous polyps have a mixed histological picture and an intermediate risk of malignant change (Fig. 8.16). Tubular and tubulo-villous adenomas may be sessile or pedunculated, single or multiple. Pedunculated polyps should be snared and removed complete (Fig. 8.17), if possible, for histological examination and to determine the presence of malignant invasion. Smaller sessile lesions can be destroyed using coagulation forceps which enable specimens to be

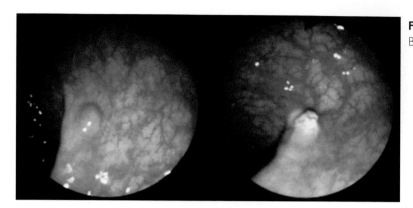

Fig. 8.18 Hot biopsy of a polyp. Before (left) and after (right) removal.

RISKS OF DEVELOPING FURTHER POLYPS	
Higher	**Lower**
large polyp multiple	small polyp single

Fig. 8.19 Risks of developing further polyps.

taken simultaneously. This is the so-called 'hot biopsy' technique (Fig. 8.18). Larger sessile lesions can be removed 'piecemeal' using a snare. The comparative risks of further polyp development are highlighted in Fig. 8.19.

SCREENING PROGRAMMES FOR COLORECTAL CANCER

There is as yet no firm evidence from controlled trials that screening of asymptomatic populations with faecal occult blood testing will reduce the morbidity and mortality of colorectal cancer. A major trial conducted in the UK is due to report in 1995.

However, follow-up programmes for individuals in high risk groups should be available with regular colonoscopic examination as the mainstay. Patients who have had adenomas should have a colonoscopy every 3 to 5 years after the colon has been cleared of polyps. Other high risk groups include those with previous colorectal carcinoma, who may develop metachronous adenomatous polyps or carcinoma, and patients with longstanding, extensive ulcerative colitis. Members of families with a high genetic risk of colorectal cancer are likely to benefit from a structured programme. Those at greatest risk are the offspring of patients with familial adenomatous polyposis, and those with hereditary non-polyposis colorectal cancer.

The potential benefits from any follow-up and screening programmes need to be weighed against the invasive nature of colonoscopy and the small but significant percentage morbidity and mortality arising from the procedure, and its acceptability to the population in general. These factors will affect the acceptance of any programme offered, and thus its effectiveness.

POINTS TO REMEMBER

- There are 20,000 deaths each year from colorectal cancer in the UK
- 25% of people who present with colorectal cancer are under 60
- Colorectal cancer is a curable disease
- Early detection gives the best chance of cure
- Only 40% of colorectal tumours present with classical symptoms
- Rectal bleeding in the absence of an anorectal lesion requires investigation of the whole colon

9. Jaundice, Alcohol and the Liver

JAUNDICE

The appearance of a yellow discoloration of the sclera and skin is one of the more dramatic signs in clinical medicine and is usually obvious to both patient and doctor (Fig. 9.1). Mild degrees of jaundice may be missed clinically unless the patient is examined in a good light. Jaundice is due to elevated levels of serum bilirubin, and is usually apparent only when the normal serum level has more than doubled. Very high carotene levels, as seen in those who eat an abnormal amount of carrots, may occasionally lead to a mistaken impression that an individual is jaundiced.

A basic understanding of bilirubin metabolism is helpful in the approach to the jaundiced patient (Fig. 9.2). Interruption of this metabolic pathway at any site may lead to jaundice (see Fig. 9.3). An increased level of unconjugated bilirubin, as seen in haemolysis, leads to increased excretion of urobilinogen, but

not bilirubin, in the urine (so-called acholuric jaundice). The more common causes of jaundice are associated with increased levels of conjugated bilirubin where bile is found in the urine.

Pathogenesis

Jaundice may be due to a number of diseases. These include viral hepatitis, extrahepatic biliary obstruction due to gall stones or pancreatic disease, metastatic

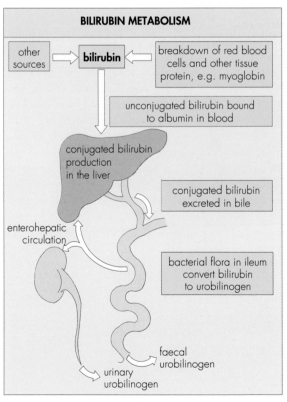

Fig. 9.2 Normal pathway of bilirubin metabolism. Conjugated bilirubin is water soluble. Some is resorbed from the bowel as urobilinogen and is predominantly re-excreted in bile with small amounts excreted in urine.

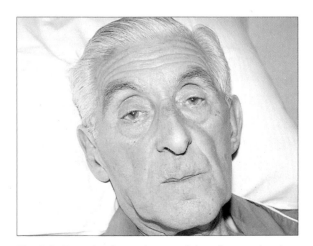

Fig. 9.1 Typical yellow sclerae and skin of a jaundiced patient

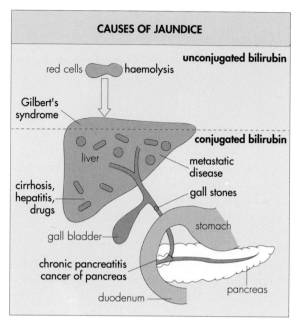

CAUSES OF JAUNDICE

red cells — haemolysis — unconjugated bilirubin

Gilbert's syndrome

liver — conjugated bilirubin

metastatic disease

cirrhosis, hepatitis, drugs

gall stones

gall bladder

stomach

chronic pancreatitis cancer of pancreas

duodenum

pancreas

Fig. 9.3 Causes of jaundice.

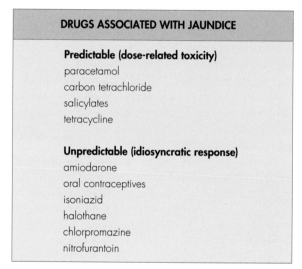

FEATURES TO NOTE IN JAUNDICE

age
occupation
drug history (prescribed, over-the-counter and illicit)
family history (jaundice, blood disorders, liver disease)
foreign travel
sexuality
alcohol consumption
previous medical history (operations, transfusions, jaundice)

Fig. 9.4 Important features in the clinical history of a jaundiced patient.

DRUGS ASSOCIATED WITH JAUNDICE

Predictable (dose-related toxicity)
paracetamol
carbon tetrachloride
salicylates
tetracycline

Unpredictable (idiosyncratic response)
amiodarone
oral contraceptives
isoniazid
halothane
chlorpromazine
nitrofurantoin

Fig. 9.5 Drugs associated with jaundice.

liver disease and chronic liver disease (especially due to alcohol and the use of certain drugs). Less commonly, jaundice may be due to haemolysis or associated with infections such as leptospirosis.

Generally, young patients are more likely to have viral hepatitis or haemolysis whilst the elderly are likely to have extrahepatic biliary obstruction from gall stones or pancreatic disease. There are less likely to be marked age differences in the case of alcohol-related disease or drug use and, here, the patient's history is of particular value.

DIAGNOSIS

Symptoms

- Prodromal symptoms
- Pruritus
- Weight loss
- Abdominal pain

It is frequently possible to establish an initial diagnosis based on the history alone (Fig. 9.4), which may be confirmed subsequently by appropriate investigations.

History

Viral Hepatitis

Viral hepatitis, particularly hepatitis A, is more common in those recently returned from endemic areas, and is often associated with the characteristic prodromal symptoms of upper abdominal discomfort, nausea, anorexia, malaise, skin rashes and arthralgia. Some patients also stop smoking. All these symptoms usually abate as the jaundice develops.

Health workers, patients with a history of multiple previous blood transfusions, intravenous drug abusers and male homosexuals are more likely to have hepatitis B or hepatitis C.

CLINICAL SIGNS IN CHRONIC LIVER DISEASE

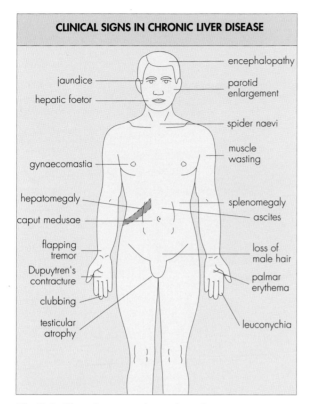

encephalopathy
jaundice
parotid enlargement
hepatic foetor
spider naevi
muscle wasting
gynaecomastia
hepatomegaly
splenomegaly
caput medusae
ascites
flapping tremor
loss of male hair
Dupuytren's contracture
palmar erythema
clubbing
testicular atrophy
leuconychia

Fig. 9.6 Clinical signs in chronic liver disease.

IMPORTANT FEATURES OF CLINICAL EXAMINATION

Evidence of liver failure
altered mental state (encephalopathy)
flapping tremor (asterixis)
hepatic foetor

Evidence of possible chronic liver disease
spider naevi, palmer erythema, white nails
muscle loss
loss of body hair, gynaecomastia, testicular atrophy
parotid enlargement
hepatomegaly
splenomegaly
prominant abdominal wall veins with flow away from the umbilicus (caput medusae)
ascites, peripheral oedema

Evidence suggesting systemic or neoplastic disease
anaemia, lymphadenopathy
a palpable gall bladder or abdominal mass

Fig. 9.7 Important features of clinical examination in the jaundiced patient.

Alcohol and Drugs

The increasing importance of alcohol cannot be overemphasized. Both chronic alcoholic liver disease and alcoholic hepatitis may cause jaundice in adults of any age. An accurate drug history is vital. The common drugs associated with jaundice are listed in Fig. 9.5. These drugs are conventionally divided into those producing a 'predictable' or cumulative dose effect and those causing jaundice due to a hypersensitivity reaction. It is not clear, however, as to why some individuals develop dose-related liver damage whilst others are unaffected.

Other Causes

In sewage workers and others exposed to potentially infected water, such as farmers and water-sports enthusiasts, leptospirosis may be considered although this is usually a more dramatic illness with severe constitutional symptoms.

Marked weight loss, particularly with abdominal pain, strongly suggests malignancy. Typically the jaundice will then be due to massive liver involve-ment with metastatic disease from primary neoplasms of the lung, stomach, colon or pancreas. (Jaundice due to bile duct obstruction is considered in Chapter 5.) A high fever, especially if associated with rigors, indicates cholangitis and biliary obstruction which is typically due to a gall stone within the common bile duct. Pruritus may be severe and is a feature of prolonged cholestasis; it is not experienced by those with raised levels of unconjugated bilirubin and therefore excludes haemolysis as the cause of jaundice.

Pregnancy may occasionally lead to jaundice. The mechanism is unknown and appropriate tests will be needed to exclude other causes of jaundice.

EXAMINATION

General physical examination seeks evidence of underlying chronic liver disease (Figs 9.6 and 9.7), other systemic or neoplastic disease and evidence of liver failure.

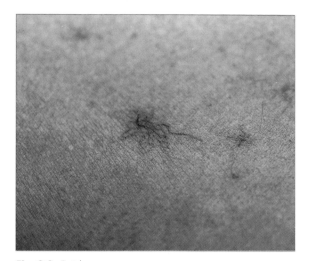

Fig. 9.8 Spider naevus.

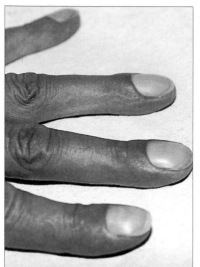

Fig. 9.10
Leuconychia and clubbing.

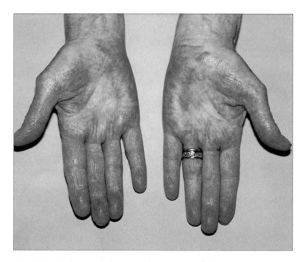

Fig. 9.9 Palmar erythema. The centre of the palm appears pale compared to the redness of the surrounding thenar and hypothenar eminences and of the tissues overlying the metacarpophalangeal joints.

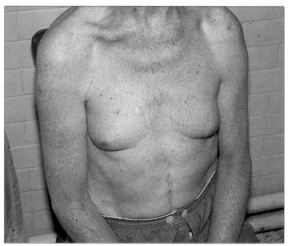

Fig. 9.11 Gynaecomastia. Often found in association with testicular atrophy and loss of body hair.

Chronic Liver Disease

Some patients with chronic liver disease have florid cutaneous manifestations of liver disease. Spider naevi (Fig. 9.8) are occasionally seen in normal individuals and during pregnancy. They are found on the upper trunk, arms and head, and it is believed that five or more are suggestive of liver disease. Spider naevi may be distinguished from other vascular lesions of the skin by a feeding arteriole which, if compressed, will cause the 'spider' to blanche. Palmar erythema (Fig. 9.9), known as 'liverpalms' in the context of liver disease, is a less specific clinical finding which may be seen in some normal individuals and in some patients with other systemic diseases. The mechanisms underlying the skin changes found in chronic liver disease, however, are unknown. White nails (leuconychia) and clubbing (Fig. 9.10) are seen in cirrhosis but are not specific.

Poorly understood endocrine changes are thought

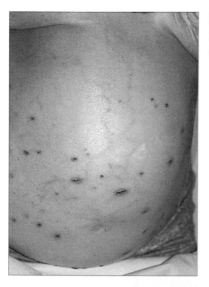

Fig. 9.12 Distended abdominal veins.

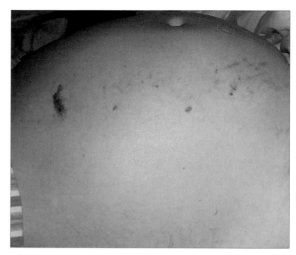

Fig. 9.14 Tense ascites in a jaundiced patient. Bruising is also present.

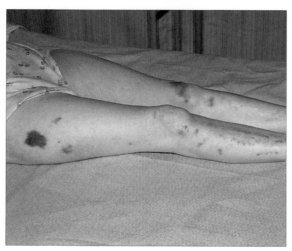

Fig. 9.13 Bruising is commonly seen in severe liver disease. It may be caused by a combination of local trauma and abnormal clotting.

to lead to loss of male body hair, testicular atrophy and gynaecomastia (Fig. 9.11). Gynaecomastia may be painful and occurs not only due to liver disease but also as a side effect of spironolactone. Prominent abdominal wall veins are seen in portal hypertension (Fig. 9.12) where they act as portosystemic collaterals. In some individuals, this is sufficiently pronounced to produce a ring of vessels around the umbilicus known as 'caput medusa'.

In those with advanced liver disease, there is often extensive bruising (Fig. 9.13). Ascites may be obvious (Fig. 9.14) and, if found with other stigmata of liver disease, are strongly suggestive of decompensated liver disease. The other main cause of ascites is intra-abdominal malignancy. At least a litre of free intra-abdominal fluid has to be present before ascites can be detected clinically, and small quantities are more often seen on ultrasound.

Hepatic encephalopathy is an important predictor of outcome and it should be specifically considered or it may be missed. The absence of hepatomegaly does not exclude chronic liver disease since the liver may become impalpable with progressive fibrotic damage.

Cholestasis

The pruritus of chronic cholestasis may be distressing and scratch marks are often seen. Xanthelasmata are an additional feature of prolonged cholestasis (see Fig. 9.15).

Other Signs

Occasionally, an hepatic bruit may be heard; this is characteristic of a tumour, such as a primary hepato-

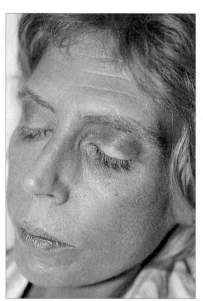

Fig. 9.15 Xanthelasmata in a woman with prolonged cholestasis due to primary biliary cirrhosis.

GILBERT'S SYNDROME
bilirubin <100µmol/l
no bile in the urine
normal transaminases
reticulocyte count less than 2%, and normal blood film

Fig. 9.17 Gilbert's syndrome.

HAEMOLYTIC ANAEMIA: COMMON CAUSES
auto-immune
associated with lymphoma or infection (e.g. mycoplasma pneumonia)
drugs (e.g. antimalarials
haemoglobinopathies (e.g. sickle-cell anaemia)
red cell enzyme deficiency (e.g. glucose-6-phosphate dehydrogenase)
hereditary spherocytosis

Fig. 9.18 Common causes of haemolytic anaemia.

INITIAL INVESTIGATIONS IN THE JAUNDICED PATIENT
full blood count and film, prothrombin time
urea and electrolytes
liver function tests—transaminase(s), alkaline phosphatase, bilirubin, total protein and albumin
hepatitis B surface antigen (HBsAg)

Fig. 9.16 Initial investigations in the jaundiced patient.

cellular carcinoma, but a bruit may also be heard in alcoholic hepatitis. A palpable gall bladder suggests extrahepatic biliary obstruction, usually due to pancreatic carcinoma.

INVESTIGATION AND MANAGEMENT

Many patients with jaundice may be appropriately investigated by their general practitioner or hospital doctor as an out-patient. This is assuming that there is ready access to the necessary investigations, which should be performed without delay. If there is evidence of either acute hepatic encephalopathy or cholangitis then urgent admission is mandatory.

Initial investigations are listed in Fig. 9.16. The results of these will determine which further tests are needed. The typical patterns of abnormality are discussed below.

Isolated Elevation of the Bilirubin Level

This is common, particularly in young patients, and is usually due to Gilbert's syndrome. The typical features of this condition are listed in Fig. 9.17. Gilbert's syndrome is often diagnosed during an intercurrent illness when the impaired hepatic handling of unconjugated bilirubin is more marked. It is entirely benign, so further investigation is not needed and the patient may be reassured. If there is uncertainty as to the diagnosis, then fasting may be used to demonstrate a further rise in serum bilirubin. Liver histology is normal and biopsy is usually avoided.

Haemolysis is a less common cause of an elevated bilirubin level, and is usually associated with normal liver enzymes. Jaundice is mild (unconjugated, and therefore there is no bilirubin in the urine) with an abnormal blood film and an increased reticulocyte count. The common causes of haemolysis are indicated in Fig. 9.18, and further management will be dictated according to the specific cause.

TYPES OF VIRAL HEPATITIS		
Type	**Blood test**	**Comment**
hepatitis A (HAV)	IgM anti-HAV	short incubation, may be epidemic
hepatitis B (HBV)	HBsAg	long incubation, usually parenteral or sexual transmission
glandular fever	IgM anti-EBV	jaundice usually mild
cytomegalovirus (CMV)	IgM anti-CMV	jaundice uncommon
hepatitis D (HDV)	anti-HDV	only in presence of acute or chronic HBV
non-A, non-B (hepatitis C and E)	anti-HCV	see text

HBsAg = hepatitis B surface antigen
EBV = Epstein–Barr virus

Fig. 9.19 Types of viral hepatitis.

Marked Elevation of Transaminase Levels

The typical finding of an 'hepatitic' illness is a rise in the levels of the serum transaminases, which can be frequently elevated by a factor of between 10 and 20 times the normal value. In a young patient, this is likely to be due to viral hepatitis. The causes and appropriate investigations are shown in Fig. 9.19. Hepatitis A is always self-limiting. Hepatitis B may become chronic in up to 5% of adults (as opposed to 90% of infants) and is then associated with chronic liver disease. A patient with chronic hepatitis B may become jaundiced either due to the deterioration of their liver disease, a superimposed viral hepatitis or because of the development of a primary hepatocellular carcinoma. Patients who fail to completely recover from the hepatitis B virus should ordinarily be referred for specialist assessment, since antiviral therapy (for example with interferon) may be appropriate. Hepatitis D occurs either with acute hepatitis B or superimposed on a background of chronic hepatitis B. It is common in Mediterranean countries and rare in the UK.

Non-A, non-B hepatitis has previously been diagnosed by exclusion and is caused by at least two different viruses. Hepatitis C causes both post-transfusion and endemic hepatitis. Recent advances have enabled serological tests for the antibody to hepatitis C to be developed, but these need to be interpreted with caution since the specificity of these tests is low, especially in patients with auto-immune chronic liver disease. The other virus previously included as non-A, non-B has been designated hepatitis E: this is a water-borne virus similar to, but serologically distinct from, hepatitis A. Other viruses, including adenoviruses, the coxsackie virus and the varicella virus may cause hepatitis as part of a more generalized illness but they only occasionally produce jaundice.

The management of acute viral hepatitis is largely symptomatic. The vast majority of patients make an uncomplicated recovery; admission to hospital, therefore, tends to be for a small number of patients with severe symptoms or social difficulty. Patients should abstain from alcohol until their liver function tests have returned to normal. Acute liver failure is rare but may occur with any type of viral hepatitis. This is an urgent situation which must be recognized since intensive care and, occasionally, liver transplantation may be needed.

If the cause of the marked elevation of transaminases remains unclear, the drug history should be reviewed again. A hepatitic blood picture may reveal the presence of chronic liver disease (see over).

FURTHER TESTS IN CHRONIC LIVER DISEASE	
Cause of disease	**Test**
auto-immune chronic active hepatitis	smooth muscle antibodies
primary biliary cirrhosis	anti-mitochondrial antibodies
haemochromatosis	serum iron and ferritin
sclerosing cholangitis	cholangiography
primary hepatocellular carcinoma	α-fetoprotein
Wilson's disease	serum copper and ceruloplasmin

Fig. 9.20 Causes of chronic liver disease and further tests that may be indicated.

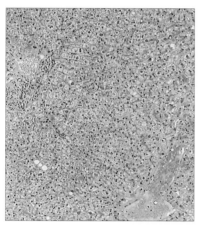

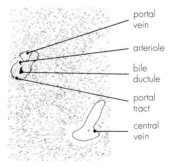

portal vein

arteriole

bile ductule

portal tract

central vein

Fig. 9.21 Normal liver. A normal portal tract containing a portal vein, arteriole and bile ductule is demonstrated, as well as the centre of the lobule containing a central vein. The hepatocytes are arranged as cords between the two structures, each cord with cell plates only one cell thick.

(the further management of this group of patients is discussed in Chapter 5). It is important to note that, in some individuals experiencing acute hepatitis, there may be a prolonged cholestatic phase after the initial 'hepatitic' illness, which may have been missed if presentation was delayed.

Where there is no evidence of obstruction to the biliary tree, the investigations carried out should be as those for a 'mixed' pattern of liver blood tests (see below).

Mixed Results in Liver Blood Tests

In these patients, the liver blood tests show both cholestatic and hepatitic features. This group usually includes most of the patients with chronic liver disease. Whilst stigmata of chronic liver disease may indeed be present many patients will have no such signs.

In addition to the specific tests for viral hepatitis already described (see Fig. 9.19), further tests that may be needed are outlined in Fig. 9.20. If the diagnosis is unclear, and a liver ultrasound has excluded biliary tract obstruction, then a percutaneous liver biopsy may be appropriate.

Liver Biopsy

Before proceeding to a liver biopsy a coagulation screen is performed. The prothrombin time should be prolonged less than 3 s more than the control, and the platelet count should be greater than $80 \times 10^9/l$. When clotting is abnormal and a liver biopsy is essential, it may still be obtained either by the transjugular route or by a modified 'plugged' percutaneous method. The liver biopsy may show a variety of changes. When compared

Cholestatic Liver Blood Tests

When initial liver function tests show marked elevation of bilirubin and alkaline phosphatase levels, together with normal or modestly elevated levels of transaminases, the pattern is described as cholestatic. The key investigation is an upper abdominal ultrasound, which will identify those patients with a dilated biliary tree due to extrahepatic biliary obstruction

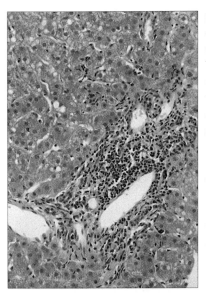

Fig. 9.22 Chronic persistent hepatitis. The portal tract near the edge of this needle biopsy contains a greatly increased number of inflammatory cells. The demarcation between the portal space and the liver substance, the limiting plate, is intact.

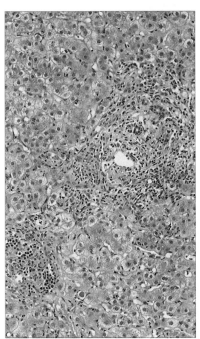

Fig. 9.23 Chronic active hepatitis. Two adjacent portal tracts are shown. Although both contain an excess of inflammatory cells, the limiting plate does not confine the changes and inflammation is spreading out. Some hepatocytes have been surrounded and look abnormal (piecemeal necrosis).

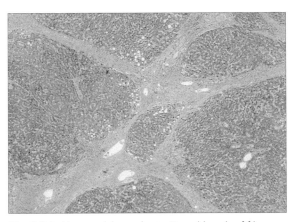

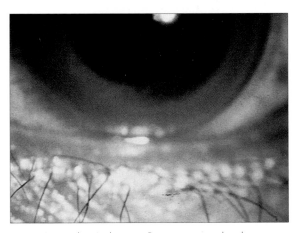

Fig. 9.24 Micronodular cirrhosis. Broad bands of fibrous tissue isolate nodules of varying size. The liver cell plates, the arrangement of cells within the lobule, do not consist of uniform, one cell thick strands but are of variable size.

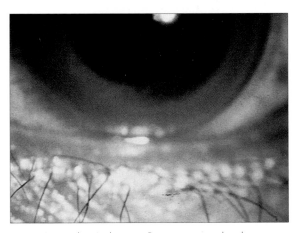

Fig. 9.25 Wilson's disease. Brown pigment has been deposited in the outermost cornea to form the characteristic Kayser–Fleischer ring

with a normal biopsy (Fig. 9.21), the inflammatory activity in chronic persistent hepatitis (Fig. 9.22) and chronic active hepatitis (Fig. 9.23) is readily appreciated. Whilst the biopsy may be diagnostic in some conditions, a particular histological pattern may be due to several possible causes (e.g. chronic active hepatitis may be auto-immune, due to chronic hepatitis B or C, associated with alcohol abuse; or due to Wilson's disease or α_1-antitrypsin deficiency). The nodules of micronodular cirrhosis are usually well seen in a liver biopsy (Fig. 9.24) but may be missed in macronodular cirrhosis. Additional information about the macroscopic appearance of the liver may be obtained by laparoscopy, which can also be used to obtain guided biopsies. In young patients, Wilson's disease needs to be excluded by using copper studies and slit-lamp eye examination (Fig. 9.25) because, although rare, it is eminently treatable.

Alcohol is by far the most common cause of chronic liver disease in Europe and the USA. A liver biopsy may show characteristic histological abnormalities but non-specific changes may be all that are seen.

Liver Ultrasound

If liver ultrasound reveals focal abnormalities, then metastatic carcinoma is the most likely diagnosis

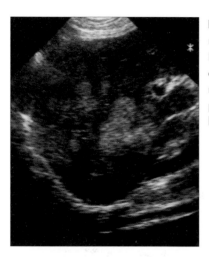

Fig. 9.26 Liver metastases. Numerous echo-dense metastases are present in the liver.

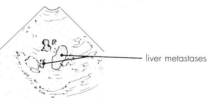

liver metastases

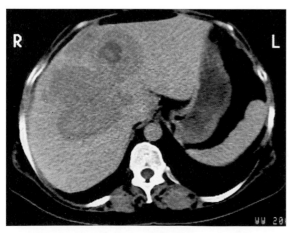

Fig. 9.27 The central portion of the liver on this CT scan is replaced by a mass which shows necrosis in its most anterior part.

(Fig. 9.26). Some lesions may be better visualized by CT scan (Fig. 9.27) which has an added advantage in that the images obtained are less operator- dependent and more readily understood by non-radiologists. Infectious causes such as amoebiasis (Fig. 9.28) and hydatid disease (Figs 9.29 and 9.30) should be considered before proceeding to liver biopsy.

When specific causes of chronic liver disease have been excluded, a diagnostic label of 'cryptogenic' liver disease may be given. Improving diagnostic techniques are reducing the numbers of patients in this group.

CONCLUSIONS

The initial assessment and investigation of jaundiced patients allows rapid identification of those with acute self-limiting viral hepatitis and those with extrahepatic biliary obstruction. Other patients require more extensive hospital-based investigations

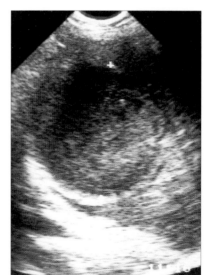

Fig. 9.28 A large abscess cavity seen on liver ultrasound. In this case it was due to amoebiasis but a pyogenic abscess may give a similar appearance.

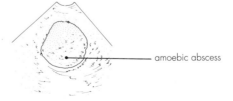

amoebic abscess

which allow a specific diagnosis to be made. Particular effort needs to be made to identify the treatable causes of chronic liver disease, such as auto-immune chronic active hepatitis, haemochromatosis and Wilson's disease. For some patients,

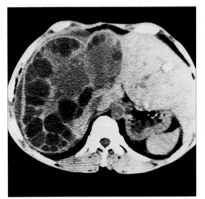

Fig. 9.29 A CT scan of the liver showing hydatid cysts. Numerous daughter cysts and the chitinous capsule can be readily seen.

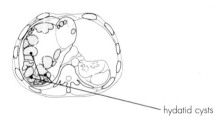

hydatid cysts

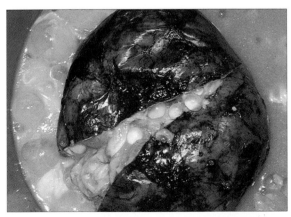

Fig. 9.30 Hydatid cysts. Rare in the UK, hydatid disease is not infrequently encountered in Eastern Europe and the Middle East. Symptoms, if any, include abdominal swelling and pain. When suspected, diagnosis should be made by non-invasive means, as fatal anaphylaxis may result from leakage of cyst fluid. Careful surgery to remove the cysts intact, as shown here, is the preferred treatment, although some antihelminthic agents may be effective.

liver transplants have become a realistic option; this emphasizes the importance of specialist assessment.

POINTS TO REMEMBER

Jaundice

- There may be no cutaneous stigmata of chronic liver disease despite advanced cirrhosis
- Hospital admission is advisable if there is acute encephalopathy, history of cholangitis, and when rapid investigation is not possible for out-patients
- Many commonly used drugs may occasionally cause jaundice: a careful drug history is vital

Acute viral hepatitis

- Treat symptomatically
- Avoid alcohol until transaminases are normal
- Hepatitis A is never chronic
- hepatitis B and C may become chronic
- always remember alcohol and drugs

Liver biopsy

- May be essential for diagnosis
- May be done as a day-case procedure in selected patients
- Ultrasound may be invaluable for biopsy of a focal lesion
- Death from haemorrhage will occur in approximately 1 in 5,000 biopsies

ALCOHOL AND THE LIVER

There are approximately 1.5 million male and 500,000 female heavy drinkers in the UK. These subjects consume, on average, more than 21 units of alcohol per week (male) or 14 units of alcohol per week (female) (see Figs 9.31 and 9.32). The unit equivalents of alcohol are shown in Fig. 9.33.

It is not surprising, with these levels of heavy drinking, that the incidence and prevalence of alcoholic liver disease are increasing. The problems of alcoholic cirrhosis were previously grossly underestimated because it was rarely cited as a cause of death as an inquest inevitably ensued. Since 1983, coroners'

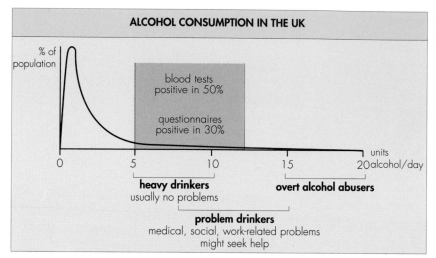

ALCOHOL CONSUMPTION IN THE UK

% of population

blood tests positive in 50%

questionnaires positive in 30%

units alcohol/day

0   5   10   15   20

heavy drinkers
usually no problems

overt alcohol abusers

problem drinkers
medical, social, work-related problems
might seek help

Fig. 9.31 Levels of alcohol consumption.

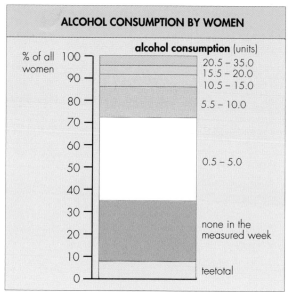

ALCOHOL CONSUMPTION BY WOMEN

alcohol consumption (units)

% of all women

100 —
90 —   20.5 – 35.0
            15.5 – 20.0
80 —   10.5 – 15.0
70 —   5.5 – 10.0
60 —
50 —   0.5 – 5.0
40 —
30 —
20 —   none in the
            measured week
10 —
0 —   teetotal

Fig. 9.32 Levels of alcohol consumption (per week): distribution of women. (Data from Wilson, P. (1980) 'OPCS Survey on Drinking in England and Wales', London: HMSO.)

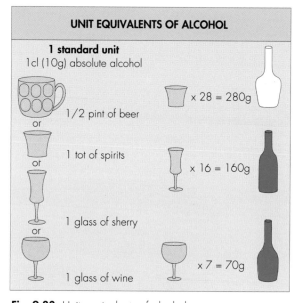

UNIT EQUIVALENTS OF ALCOHOL

1 standard unit
1cl (10g) absolute alcohol

1/2 pint of beer
or
1 tot of spirits
or
1 glass of sherry
or
1 glass of wine

x 28 = 280g

x 16 = 160g

x 7 = 70g

Fig. 9.33 Unit equivalents of alcohol.

rules have changed to allow alcohol to be certified as a cause of death and this has led to an increase in apparent deaths due to alcoholic cirrhosis.

Alcoholic liver disease in its various forms —fatty liver (Fig. 9.34), hepatitis cirrhosis (fig. 9.35) — is extremely common, but the true problem can only be established by percutaneous liver biopsy being performed on all heavy drinkers. Between 10% and 15% of beds, in the average district general hospital gastroenterology unit, are occupied by patients with

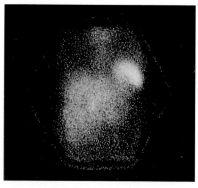

Fig. 9.34
Isotope scan of a fatty liver.

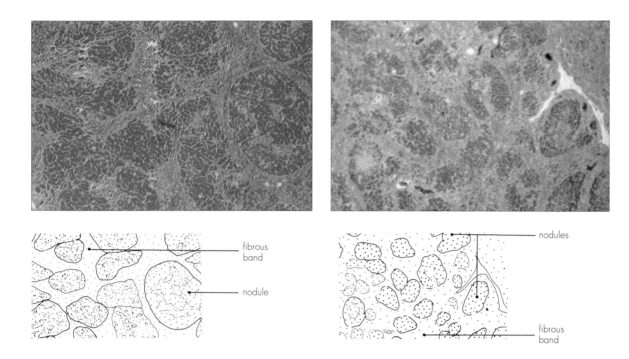

Fig. 9.35 Micronodular cirrhosis showing total destruction of the architecture and replacement by regenerative nodules and fibrous bands. H & E stain, x30 (left). Masson trichome stain, x12 (right).

alcoholic liver disease. The only treatment for this condition is abstention from alcohol, but unfortunately cirrhosis, once established, is irreversible. Attention is therefore focused on the early detection of alcoholic liver disease, and particular interest is focused on the factors which may lead to an increased susceptibility to alcoholic liver damage (Fig. 9.36).

History

There is little difficulty in the diagnosis of patients who are prepared to admit their true levels of alcohol consumption. All too often, however, the history may either be inadequately taken by the doctor or patients lie about their drinking habits. In these circumstances, corroborative evidence from close relatives may be required or objective measurements of alcohol abuse, such as blood alcohol or urinary alcohol levels, may have to be relied upon.

Various haematological and biochemical measures have been used to detect alcoholic liver disease (Figs 9.37 and 9.38), but these may produce either false

INCREASED SUSCEPTIBILITY TO ALCOHOLIC LIVER DAMAGE
female
family history
obesity

Fig. 9.36 Factors which determine susceptibility to alcoholic liver damage.

DETECTION OF HEAVY DRINKING
blood tests
questionnaires
non-specific indicators

Fig. 9.37 Detection of heavy drinking.

SCREENING TESTS
γ-glutamyl transpeptidase
mean corpuscular volume
blood alcohol
urine alcohol

Fig. 9.38 Screening tests for alcoholic liver disease.

positive or false negative results. The search is still on for specific biochemical or haematological indicators of alcohol abuse.

In the history, careful attention should be given to the frequency of drinking, the types of drink imbibed, the duration of drinking, alcohol-free periods, family history of alcohol abuse and other important social factors, such as employment and marital status. The type of alcohol taken is of no importance, in relation to the severity of liver damaged incurred.

DIAGNOSIS

On examination, although the typical heavy drinker, classically, is plethoric with a bulbous, swollen nose, and obese, the typical signs of alcoholic liver disease do not appear unless the patient has advanced alcoholic hepatitis or alcoholic cirrhosis. It cannot be diagnosed on the basis of blood tests, which may be normal, even with advanced liver disease. The gold standard for diagnosis is liver biopsy. For the signs of alcoholic liver disease, see Figs 9.8, 9.9, 9.10 and 9.14.

EXAMINATION

Examination should be focused on eliciting the physical signs shown in the figures above, but more subtle signs should be sought, such as spider naevi (which may only be present on the fingers) and leuconychia. There may be no signs at all, even in advanced cases.

TREATMENT

There is no treatment for alcoholic liver disease apart from abstention from alcohol, although many, many therapeutic regimes have been tried. The use of B vitamins is often no better than placebo, and there is no evidence that anti-thyroid drugs, such as propylthiouracil, are of long-term benefit. Treatment of acute alcoholic hepatitis with intravenous amino-acid solutions and/or corticosteroids is still under clinical trial. The only treatment that appears to be effective

in managing the final stages of alcoholic cirrhosis is liver transplantation, which is now considered for patients who have demonstrated their ability to abstain for more than six months.

PROGNOSIS

Patients with a fatty liver excluding perivenular fibrosis should expect full recovery of their liver, provided they abstain from alcohol completely. Unfortunately, once perivenular fibrosis is established, the progression to cirrhosis may occur even if patients stop drinking. Clearly progression is faster when patients continue to imbibe alcohol.

Alcoholic hepatitis almost inevitably leads to cirrhosis and, once established, it cannot be reversed.

In view of the rather gloomy prognosis of alcoholic liver disease the key is early prevention. This is primarily an educational undertaking but there are great difficulties in convincing healthy subjects that their alcohol consumption, if they are free of symptoms may be dangerous.

The identification of susceptible individuals is paramount and educating them in a convincing and productive manner is of importance. Factors which determine an individual's susceptibility to alcohol remain unclear, but there is almost certainly a genetic basis that is also gender related. Unfortunately, by the time the disease is clinically apparent liver disease is often irreversible.

POINTS TO REMEMBER

- A qualitative drinking history is not sufficient
- Regular heavy drinking is dangerous
- Women are twice as susceptible to alcohol
- Cirrhosis is irreversible
- Heavy drinkers may have normal liver function tests

10. Gall Stones

INTRODUCTION

Approximately 1 litre of bile per day is secreted into the bile ducts. Bile is concentrated within the gall bladder, where more than 80% of the water and electrolytes are resorbed. After eating, and under the influence of cholecystokinin, the gall bladder contracts and bile is secreted into the duodenum. The primary bile acids, such as cholic acid and chenodeoxycholic acid, are converted by bowel bacteria to secondary bile acids before being resorbed (Fig. 10.1). This enterohepatic circulation of bile acids may occur up to ten times per day.

The formation of gall stones is incompletely understood, but any change in bile composition, gall bladder function or infection within the biliary tree increases the risk of their formation.

Epidemiology

Gall stones remain a major cause of morbidity in the West, and cholecystectomy is still the most common major abdominal operation in developed countries.

Types of Gall Stone

The vast majority of gall stones, in the UK and other western countries, are predominantly composed of cholesterol alone or cholesterol plus bile pigment and calcium (mixed stones). Pigment stones are less common and are often radio-opaque (see Fig. 10.2). These types of stone are considered separately below.

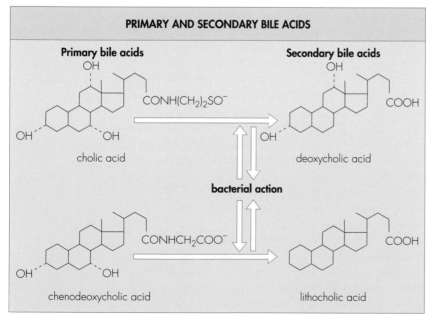

Fig. 10.1 Structures of primary and secondary bile acids.

TYPES OF GALL STONES		
	Cholesterol stones	Pigment stones
frequency in UK (%)	80	20
radiopaque (%)	15	60

Fig. 10.2 Types of gall stone.

RISK FACTORS ASSOCIATED WITH CHOLESTEROL GALL STONE FORMATION	
age	progressively more frequent
sex	women have double the incidence, especially under the age of 50
obesity	increased cholesterol synthesis and excretion
diet	reduced incidence in vegetarians; cholesterol reducing diets lead to increased gall stone formation
drugs	clofibrate, cholestyramine, oral contraceptives
also	family history, ileal resection, liver disease

Fig. 10.3 Risk factors associated with cholesterol gall stone formation.

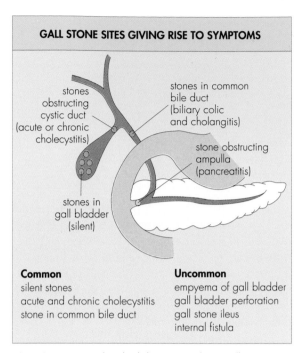

| GALL STONE SITES GIVING RISE TO SYMPTOMS |

Common
silent stones
acute and chronic cholecystitis
stone in common bile duct

Uncommon
empyema of gall bladder
gall bladder perforation
gall stone ileus
internal fistula

Fig. 10.4 Sites within the biliary tree where gall stones may lead to the manifestation of symptoms.

Cholesterol Gall Stones

Cholesterol within bile is derived both from the diet and from cholesterol synthesized by the liver. Cholesterol synthesis is rate-limited by the enzyme β-hydroxy-methylglutaryl-CoA (HMGCoA) reductase. Cholesterol is insoluble in water: it is suspended in bile as micelles of cholesterol, bile salts and phospholipid. It is thought that cholesterol stones are likely to form when bile becomes supersaturated with cholesterol, relative to the amounts of bile salts and phospholipid. Cholesterol is also transported within bile by the formation of vesicles with phospholipid, without bile acids. Supersaturated bile clearly does not inevitably lead to cholesterol stone formation since healthy individuals often have supersaturated bile during fasting.

The major risk factors for cholesterol gall stone formation are shown in Fig. 10.3. They are particularly common in western countries, but the highest incidence is found amongst Native Americans.

Pigment Gall Stones

These are small and contain less than 25% cholesterol. They are particularly associated with chronic haemolysis, which leads to increased bilirubin production. Pigment stones are also usually found within the biliary tree with any condition that leads to biliary stasis, such as sclerosing cholangitis or bile duct strictures. Parasitic infections due to the roundworm, *Ascaris lumbricoides,* or the liver fluke, *Clonorchis sinensis,* are important causes of pigment stone formation in the Far East.

Pathogenesis

The Natural History of Gall Stones

Many gall stones are 'silent' and found incidentally at surgery or during investigations for unrelated conditions. Symptoms are caused by the migration of stones within the biliary tree (Fig. 10.4). Obstruction

IMAGING OF GALL STONES AND THE BILIARY TRACT

plain abdominal X-ray
oral cholecystogram
ultrasound
CT scan
isotope scan (HIDA)
endoscopic retrograde cholangiopancreatography (ERCP)
percutaneous transhepatic cholangiography

Fig. 10.5 Imaging of gall stones and the biliary tract.

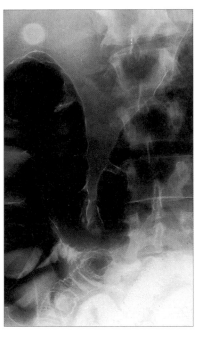

Fig. 10.6 A solitary calcified gall stone is noted during a barium meal examination.

to the cystic duct leads to secondary infection of the static bile within the gall bladder and thus to acute or chronic cholecystitis. If stones pass into the common bile duct, they may pass spontaneously into the duodenum or may obstruct the duct to give biliary colic, often with jaundice and cholangitis. Gall bladder perforation into the peritoneum or into the bowel with fistula formation is rare. Gall stone ileus is also uncommon. The passage of a stone through the ampulla of Vater may precipitate attacks of acute pancreatitis.

DIAGNOSIS

Symptoms and signs of acute cholecystitis

- Pain in the right hypochondrium
- Murphy's sign
- Nausea and vomiting
- Tachypnoea
- Fever
- Epigastric discomfort

Acute Cholecystitis

Typical features are pain in the right hypochondrium, radiating to the back and shoulder. Nausea and vomiting are frequent. Patients are ill with tachypnoea, fever, tenderness in the right hypochondrium, which becomes worse on inspiration (Murphy's sign), and often there is rebound tenderness. Other acute abdominal emergencies will need to be excluded. Treatment is with intravenous fluids and

antibiotics. Cholecystectomy is usually performed within a few days or after two months.

Chronic Cholecystitis

This is a difficult clinical diagnosis to make because the symptom complex of nausea, right hypochondrial pain and epigastric discomfort is non-specific. Unless there is a clear history of episodic biliary colic or acute cholecystitis, it is just as likely that functional bowel disease may be causing the symptoms.

INVESTIGATIONS

Imaging of the Biliary Tree and Gall Stones

A variety of methods are available (Fig. 10.5). Ten per cent of gall stones are radiopaque and may therefore be identified by a plain abdominal X-ray (Fig. 10.6). An oral cholecystogram will allow detection of more than 95% of gall bladder stones, providing the patient is not jaundiced (see Fig. 10.7). Ultrasound is being increasingly used instead of oral cholecystography as gall stones cast a characteristic acoustic shadow (Fig. 10.8). Ultrasound is equally accurate, when compared with an oral cholecytogram, but very operator-dependent; it allows the simultaneous examination of the liver, biliary tree and pancreas and is particularly useful in the jaundiced patient.

CT scanning is rarely used for the diagnosis of gall stones but allows the density of the stones to be assessed if oral dissolution therapy is being considered (see opposite). Isotope scanning, using technetium-labelled HIDA (2,6-dimethylphenylcarbamoyl-methyliminodiacetic acid), is useful for the diagnosis of acute cholecystitis. The isotope is concentrated in the bile and followed into the duodenum. If the cystic duct is obstructed, the gall bladder fails to opacify.

Endoscopic (ERCP) or percutaneous transhepatic cholangiography are particularly useful for defining the anatomy of the biliary tree. Where an obstruction is revealed, with dilatation of the bile ducts confirmed by ultrasound, then either technique may be used and the choice will be influenced by the availability of local expertise. If there is no dilatation of the biliary tree then endoscopic cholangiography is preferable. ERCP is particularly useful for the identification of gall stones within the common bile duct (Fig. 10.9).

TREATMENT

There are a variety of management options both for stones within the gall bladder and those within the bile ducts (Fig. 10.10).

Gall Stones within the Gall Bladder

In most individuals, 'silent' gall bladder stones should not be removed since only 10% will develop symptoms within 5 years. Although gall stones are

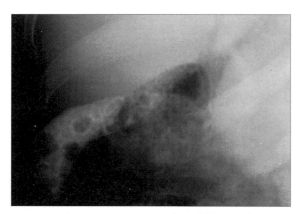

Fig. 10.7 The numerous large and small filling defects seen on this cholecystogram are gall stones. During an oral cholecystogram a fatty meal is given to stimulate contraction of the gall bladder and, if successful, this often makes the stones more apparent.

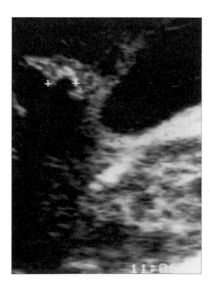

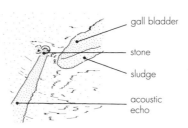

Fig. 10.8 This ultrasound shows a gall stone in the neck of the gall bladder. The acoustic echo of the stone is clearly seen as well as the contents of the gall bladder with a layer of biliary sludge.

gall bladder

stone

sludge

acoustic echo

associated with gall bladder cancer, the risks of prophylactic surgery outweigh its benefits.

Medical

The 'medical' treatment of gall stones, using oral bile acid therapy, is confined to those individuals with radiolucent stones that are smaller than 1.5 cm in diameter within a functioning gall bladder. A CT scan may be used to assess stone density and to exclude those stones which are heavily calcified. Unfortunately, these restrictions mean that oral dissolution therapy is of value in less than 30% of patients. The main side effect of chenodeoxycholic acid is diarrhoea, but tolerance may be improved by using a lower dose in combination with a low dose of ursodeoxycholic acid. Unfortunately, treatment is prolonged (2 years or more) with the recurrence of stones at a rate of 10% per annum.

Cholecystectomy

Cholecystectomy remains the 'gold standard' against which other methods of treating gall stones must be judged. Unlike the procedures described below, the gall bladder is removed thus preventing recurrence. The operation is safe, with a mortality rate of less than 0.1% in patients under 50 years of age. The main disadvantage is that of a muscle-splitting incision, which can mean considerable morbidity. Also, the majority of individuals may be away from work for between four and six weeks after a relatively long hospital stay. In recent years mini-cholecystectomy, using a much smaller incision, has begun to be practised.

Laparoscopic Cholecystectomy

The management of gall bladder stones has been revolutionized by the advent of laparoscopic cholecystectomy. The operation can be performed with a hospital stay of less than 24 hours, and individuals can return to work within a few days. The technique is popular both with patients and hospital managers. Prospective studies comparing the laparoscopic and standard techniques have not been done and, in view of the almost immediate acceptance of the operation, it appears unlikely that a truly prospective study will be performed. Recent data from both

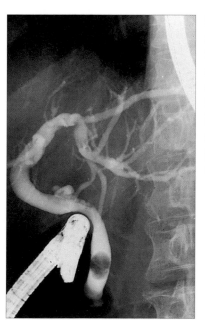

Fig. 10.9 A single gall stone in the distal common bile duct is shown as a filling defect by ERCP. The patient had previously had a cholecystectomy.

MANAGEMENT OPTIONS FOR GALL STONES

Within the gall bladder

no action

'medical' dissolution with oral bile acids

cholecystectomy
   standard
   'mini'
   laparoscopic

transhepatic dissolution

sub-hepatic, transperitoneal stone extraction

short-wave lithotripsy (ESWL)

Within the bile ducts

ERCP with sphincterotomy and stone extraction

mechanical lithotripsy

short-wave lithotripsy

ultrasound lithotripsy

laser lithotripsy

biliary endoprosthesis to prevent stone impaction

Fig. 10.10 Management options for gall stones.

ACCESS SITES FOR LAPAROSCOPIC CHOLECYSTECTOMY

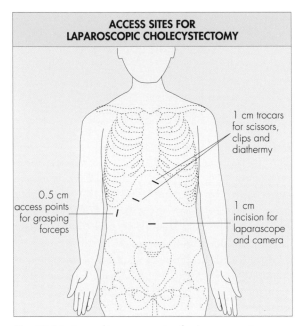

1 cm trocars for scissors, clips and diathermy

0.5 cm access points for grasping forceps

1 cm incision for laparascope and camera

Fig. 10.11 Sites of instrumentation for laparoscopic cholecystectomy.

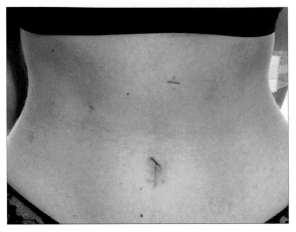

Fig. 10.12 The abdomen four weeks after laparoscopic cholecystectomy.

UNCERTAINTIES OF LAPAROSCOPIC CHOLECYSTECTOMY

should an intra-operative cholangiogram be performed for every patient ?

are lasers of any additional benefit for dissection, or are they hazardous ?

what are the exact contraindications of the procedure ?

Fig. 10.13 Uncertainties of laparoscopic cholecystectomy.

Europe and the USA indicate that the morbidity and mortality of laparoscopic cholecystectomy is very low and compares favourably with standard open cholecystectomy.

Patients selected for laparoscopic cholecystectomy should be fit enough to undergo standard cholecystectomy, if there are likely to be operative difficulties. Laparoscopic cholecystectomy is performed using four areas of abdominal access (Fig. 10.11). A standard subumbilical approach is used for the laparoscope, with access for the other instruments as shown.

The rapid acceptance of the technique has created some initial difficulties. It takes longer to perform than open cholecystectomy; it has created problems for surgical training and there is still a shortage of the appropriate instruments in some centres.

It is not surprising, in view of the short hospital stay and excellent cosmetic results (Fig. 10.12), that the procedure is requested by many patients. Even so, several important questions remain unanswered, prospective studies will be needed to answer them (Fig. 10.13), and the precise role of this exciting new procedure has not yet been defined.

Other Approaches

Extracorporeal shock wave lithotripsy can now be used to fragment gall stones. Modern machines do not require the use of general anaesthesia or water baths. Unfortunately, the machines are expensive and less than 20% of patients are suitable. Not only must the stones be radiolucent in a functioning gall bladder, but they need to be less than 3 cm in size and only up to three in number. Complications can arise as fragments pass through the bile ducts, so treatment tends to be combined with the administration of oral bile acids for several months.

Gall stones may be dissolved *in situ* using methy *tert*-butyl ether (MTBE), which is instilled via a catheter. The latter is inserted under ultrasound control, transhepatically, into the gall bladder (Fig. 10.14). Cholesterol stones will dissolve in less than 24 hours but the procedure is tedious. Duodenal

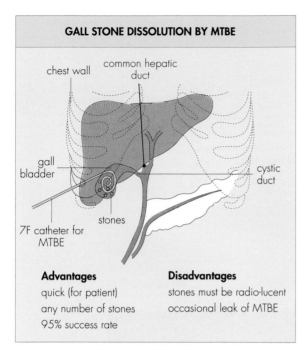

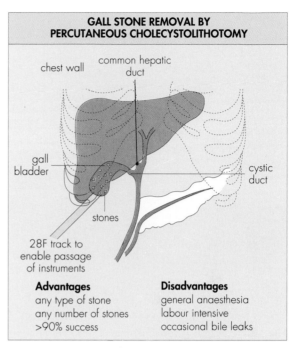

Fig. 10.14 Dissolution of gall bladder stones by methyl *tert*-butyl (MTBE).

Fig. 10.15 Removed of gall stones by percutaneous cholecystolithotomy.

leakage of the solvent has to avoided since haemolysis, duodenitis and anaesthesia may develop. An alternative is to approach the gall bladder transperitoneally and to dilate a track through which a nephroscope may be inserted and through which stones can be extracted after crushing, if necessary (Fig. 10.15). The advantage of the latter technique is that any type or number of stones may be removed, but it is labour intensive, may have significant complications and requires anaesthesia.

Gall Stones within the Bile Ducts (Choledocholithiasis)

These are usually treated either by cholecystectomy and surgical exploration of the duct or by ERCP and stone extraction. The latter technique is clearly appropriate where there has been a previous cholecystectomy or if the patient is frail or elderly. Endoscopic sphincterotomy consists of incising the papilla, and the surrounding distal common bile duct, by the use of diathermy. A good understanding of the basic anatomy is essential (Fig. 10.16). Typical

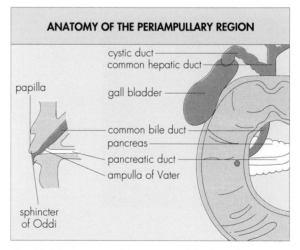

Fig. 10.16 Anatomy of the common bile duct. The common hepatic duct joins the cystic duct to form the common bile duct which traverses the head of the pancreas and empties into the duodenum through the ampulla of Vater. This intraduodenal portion of the common bile duct is enveloped by circular and longitudinal smooth muscle fibres forming the sphincter of Oddi. The papilla is usually located in the second portion of the duodenum in its posteromedial wall.

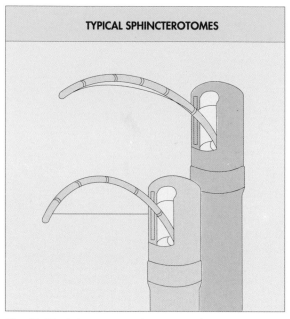

TYPICAL SPHINCTEROTOMES

Fig. 10.17 Side-viewing endoscopes with a sphincterotome in the 'relaxed' position for cannulating the ampulla (upper) and in the 'bowed' position for sphincterotomy (lower).

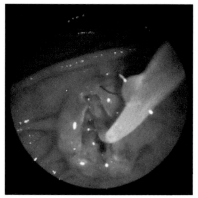

Fig. 10.18 A complete sphincterotomy incision with the sphincterotome still *in situ*.

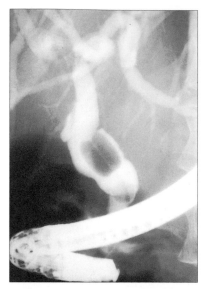

Fig. 10.19 Balloon extraction of a common bile duct stone. The balloon is fully inflated within the duct and situated above the stone.

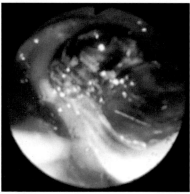

Fig. 10.20 A gall stone emerging from the papilla as a balloon is withdrawn from the common bile duct.

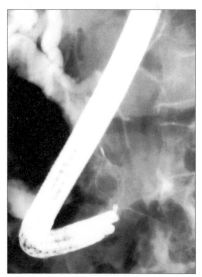

Fig. 10.21 Radiograph demonstrating a lithotriptor in use. A large stone is trapped inside the wires. By manipulating the handle of the lithotriptor, a crushing force is generated. The stone is crushed and thus is more easily extracted.

sphincterotomes are shown in Fig. 10.17, and the method of sphincterotomy is shown in Fig. 10.18. After sphincterotomy, stones may be extracted by inflating a balloon within the bile duct above the stone (Fig. 10.19) and then withdrawing the balloon so that the stone is pulled into the bowel lumen (Fig. 10.20). An alternative method of stone extraction is that effected by the use of a dormier basket.

If the stones cannot be extracted after an endo-scopic sphincterotomy they may be crushed using a mechanical lithotriptor within the duct (Fig. 10.21) or fragmented by sound waves or by a laser. An experimental system using a 'mother and baby' endoscope system (an endoscope within the standard duodeno-scope that is inserted into the common bile duct) has been evolved to facilitate these fragmentation methods, but it is still being evaluated. If duct stones cannot be removed, acceptable drainage may be ensured by the placement of pigtail biliary stents (Fig. 10.22). Again, these are particularly suitable for elderly, frail patients.

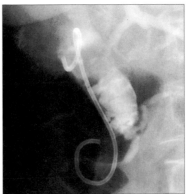

Fig. 10.22 The common bile duct stone seen here was large and difficult to extract. An endoprosthesis was placed to facilitate biliary drainage and to prevent stone impaction. The large stone can be seen in the distal portion of the bile duct.

POINTS TO REMEMBER

- Incidence increases with age
- In western countries, 15% of men and nearly 20% of women will have gall bladder stones by the age of 60
- More than 80% of stones are clinically 'silent'
- Most silent gall stones need no treatment
- Vague upper abdominal symptoms are likely to be due to functional bowel disease, even if gall stones are present
- Consider cholecystectomy in selected patients such as young diabetics, and those with calcified gall bladders and gall stones found incidentally at laparotomy

Laparascopic cholecystectomy

- requires more operating time
- allows a much shorter hopsital stay
- has reduced morbidity
- facilities for therapeutic ERCP should be available
- is still being evaluated

Endoscopic sphincterotomy

- coagulation should be normal
- has a complication rate of about 5% (haemorrhage, perforation, pancreatitis) with a mortality rate of approximately 1%
- should be performed when the risks of surgery exceed the risks of sphincterotomy.

Index